2nd Edition: The Impact of ENT Diseases in Social Life

2nd Edition: The Impact of ENT Diseases in Social Life

Editors

Francesco Gazia
Bruno Galletti
Gay-Escoda Cosme
Francesco Ciodaro
Rocco Bruno

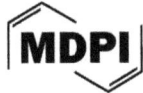 Basel • Beijing • Wuhan • Barcelona • Belgrade • Novi Sad • Cluj • Manchester

Editors

Francesco Gazia
Unit of Otorhinolaryngology
University of Messina
Messina
Italy

Bruno Galletti
Unit of Otorhinolaryngology
University of Messina
Messina
Italy

Gay-Escoda Cosme
Oral Surgery
University of Barcelona
Barcelona
Spain

Francesco Ciodaro
Division for
Otorhinolaryngology
University of Messina
Messina
Italy

Rocco Bruno
Unit of Otorhinolaryngology
University of Messina
Messina
Italy

Editorial Office
MDPI
St. Alban-Anlage 66
4052 Basel, Switzerland

This is a reprint of articles from the Special Issue published online in the open access journal *International Journal of Environmental Research and Public Health* (ISSN 1660-4601) (available at: www.mdpi.com/journal/ijerph/special_issues/2ndENT_Diseases).

For citation purposes, cite each article independently as indicated on the article page online and as indicated below:

Lastname, A.A.; Lastname, B.B. Article Title. *Journal Name* **Year**, *Volume Number*, Page Range.

ISBN 978-3-7258-0034-6 (Hbk)
ISBN 978-3-7258-0033-9 (PDF)
doi.org/10.3390/books978-3-7258-0033-9

© 2024 by the authors. Articles in this book are Open Access and distributed under the Creative Commons Attribution (CC BY) license. The book as a whole is distributed by MDPI under the terms and conditions of the Creative Commons Attribution-NonCommercial-NoDerivs (CC BY-NC-ND) license.

Contents

Salvatore Martellucci, Andrea Stolfa, Andrea Castellucci, Giulio Pagliuca, Veronica Clemenzi and Valentina Terenzi et al.
Recovery of Regular Daily Physical Activities Prevents Residual Dizziness after Canalith Repositioning Procedures
Reprinted from: *Int. J. Environ. Res. Public Health* **2022**, *19*, 490, doi:10.3390/ijerph19010490 . . . **1**

Carmelo Saraniti, Gaetano Patti and Barbara Verro
Sulcus Vocalis and Benign Vocal Cord Lesions: Is There Any Relationship?
Reprinted from: *Int. J. Environ. Res. Public Health* **2023**, *20*, 5654, doi:10.3390/ijerph20095654 . . . **10**

I-An Shih, Chung-Y. Hsu, Tsai-Chung Li and Shuu-Jiun Wang
Benign Paroxysmal Positional Vertigo Is Associated with an Increased Risk for Migraine Diagnosis: A Nationwide Population-Based Cohort Study
Reprinted from: *Int. J. Environ. Res. Public Health* **2023**, *20*, 3563, doi:10.3390/ijerph20043563 . . . **20**

Giuseppe Alberti, Daniele Portelli and Cosimo Galletti
Healthcare Professionals and Noise-Generating Tools: Challenging Assumptions about Hearing Loss Risk
Reprinted from: *Int. J. Environ. Res. Public Health* **2023**, *20*, 6520, doi:10.3390/ijerph20156520 . . . **32**

Aleksander Zwierz, Krzysztof Domagalski, Krystyna Masna and Paweł Burduk
Siblings' Risk of Adenoid Hypertrophy: A Cohort Study in Children
Reprinted from: *Int. J. Environ. Res. Public Health* **2023**, *20*, 2910, doi:10.3390/ijerph20042910 . . . **47**

Giulio Pagliuca, Veronica Clemenzi, Andrea Stolfa, Salvatore Martellucci, Antonio Greco and Marco de Vincentiis et al.
Use of Irrigation Device for Duct Dilatation during Sialendoscopy
Reprinted from: *Int. J. Environ. Res. Public Health* **2022**, *19*, 14830, doi:10.3390/ijerph192214830 . **59**

Melysa Fitriana and Chyi-Huey Bai
Hearing Problems in Indonesia: Attention to Hypertensive Adults
Reprinted from: *Int. J. Environ. Res. Public Health* **2022**, *19*, 9222, doi:10.3390/ijerph19159222 . . . **64**

Carmelo Saraniti, Francesco Ciodaro, Cosimo Galletti, Salvatore Gallina and Barbara Verro
Swallowing Outcomes in Open Partial Horizontal Laryngectomy Type I and Endoscopic Supraglottic Laryngectomy: A Comparative Study
Reprinted from: *Int. J. Environ. Res. Public Health* **2022**, *19*, 8050, doi:10.3390/ijerph19138050 . . . **75**

So Young Kim, Dae Myoung Yoo, Soo-Hwan Byun, Chanyang Min, Ji Hee Kim and Mi Jung Kwon et al.
Association between Temporomandibular Joint Disorder and Weight Changes: A Longitudinal Follow-Up Study Using a National Health Screening Cohort
Reprinted from: *Int. J. Environ. Res. Public Health* **2021**, *18*, 11793, doi:10.3390/ijerph182211793 . **84**

Carmelo Saraniti, Barbara Verro, Francesco Ciodaro and Francesco Galletti
Oncological Outcomes of Primary vs. Salvage OPHL Type II: A Systematic Review
Reprinted from: *Int. J. Environ. Res. Public Health* **2022**, *19*, 1837, doi:10.3390/ijerph19031837 . . . **94**

So Young Kim, Dae Myoung Yoo, Chanyang Min and Hyo Geun Choi
Increased Risk of Neurodegenerative Dementia after Benign Paroxysmal Positional Vertigo
Reprinted from: *Int. J. Environ. Res. Public Health* **2021**, *18*, 10553, doi:10.3390/ijerph181910553 . **105**

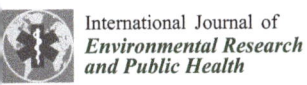

Article

Recovery of Regular Daily Physical Activities Prevents Residual Dizziness after Canalith Repositioning Procedures

Salvatore Martellucci [1], Andrea Stolfa [1,2,*], Andrea Castellucci [3], Giulio Pagliuca [1], Veronica Clemenzi [1,2], Valentina Terenzi [1,4], Pasquale Malara [5], Giuseppe Attanasio [6], Francesco Gazia [7] and Andrea Gallo [1,3]

1. ENT Unit, Ospedale "Santa Maria Goretti", Azienda USL Latina, 04100 Latina, Italy; dott.martellucci@gmail.com (S.M.); dott.giuliopagliuca@gmail.com (G.P.); veronica.clemenzi@gmail.com (V.C.); terenzivalentina@gmail.com (V.T.); andrea.gallo@uniroma1.it (A.G.)
2. ENT Clinic, Department of Sense Organs, Sapienza University of Rome, 00185 Rome, Italy
3. ENT Unit, Department of Surgery, Arcispedale Santa Maria Nuova, AUSL—IRCCS, 43123 Reggio Emilia, Italy; andrea.castellucci@ausl.re.it
4. Department of Odontostomatological e Maxillofacial Sciences, Sapienza University of Rome, 00185 Rome, Italy
5. Audiology & Vestibology Service, Centromedico Bellinzona, 6500 Bellinzona, Switzerland; pasmalara@gmail.com
6. Head and Neck Department, Umberto I Policlinic of Rome, 00185 Rome, Italy; giuseppe.attanasio@uniroma1.it
7. Unit of Otorhinolaryngology, Department of Adult and Development Age Human Pathology "Gaetano Barresi", University of Messina, 98124 Messina, Italy; ssgazia@gmail.com
* Correspondence: stolfa.an@gmail.com; Tel.: +39-3487942918

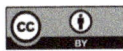

Abstract: Objective: Residual dizziness is a disorder of unknown pathophysiology, which may occur after repositioning procedures for benign paroxysmal positional vertigo. This study evaluates the relationship between regular daily physical activity and the development of residual dizziness after treatment for benign paroxysmal positional vertigo. Study Design: Prospective observational cohort study. Setting: Academic university hospital. Methods: Seventy-one patients admitted with benign paroxysmal positional vertigo involving the posterior semicircular canal were managed with Epley's procedure. Three days after successful treatment, the patients underwent a telephone interview to investigate vertigo relapse. If the patients no longer complained of vertigo, they were asked about symptoms consistent with residual dizziness. Subsequently, they were asked about the recovery of physical activities they regularly performed prior to the onset of vertigo. Results: Sixty-nine patients (age: 57.79 ± 15.05) were enrolled: five (7.24%) reported vertigo relapse whereas twenty-one of sixty-four non-relapsed patients (32.81%) reported residual dizziness. A significant difference in the incidence of residual dizziness was observed considering the patients' age ($p = 0.0003$). Of the non-relapsed patients, 46 (71.88%) recovered their regular dynamic daily activities after treatment and 9 (19.57%) reported residual dizziness, while 12 of the 18 patients (66.67%) who did not resume daily activity reported residual symptoms ($p = 0.0003$). A logistic regression analysis showed a significant association between daily activity resumption and lack of residual dizziness (OR: 14.01, 95% CI limits 3.14–62.47; $p = 0.001$). Conclusions: Regardless of age, the resumption of regular daily physical activities is associated with a lack of residual dizziness.

Keywords: residual dizziness; benign paroxysmal positional vertigo (BPPV); vertigo; canalithiasis; canalith repositioning procedure (CRP)

1. Introduction

Benign paroxysmal positional vertigo (BPPV) is the most common vestibular complaint, consisting of short-lasting vertigo spells triggered by head position changes. BPPV affects both utricular macula and one or more semicircular canals as the most accredited pathophysiology is the displacement of otoconial matter from the utricle to the involved canal. Free-floating otoconia modify endolymphatic flows and cupular responses during head movements, resulting in positional vertigo and nystagmus [1,2].

BPPV can be classified, in clinical practice, according to the affected semicircular canal (SC) and the involved arm, as follows [1,2]:

- Posterior Semicircular Canal (PSC) BPPV: Geotropic and apogeotropic variants
- Horizontal Semicircular Canal (HSC) BPPV: Geotropic and apogeotropic variants
- Anterior Semicircular Canal (ASC) BPPV
- Multicanal BPPV

The involvement of a single SC represents the most frequent condition, although BPPV might simultaneously affect more SCs on one or both sides. PSC BPPV is the most frequent variant (80–90%), whereas cases involving the HSC and ASC account for 10–20% and 3% of all BPPVs, respectively [3]. In addition, canalith jam (CJ) is an uncommon variant of vestibular lithiasis [4–6].

The diagnosis of BPPV concerning the affected ear and the involved canal and arm is commonly made by performing positioning tests, also known as diagnostic maneuvers. The tests work by gravity and inertial/centrifugal forces, which bend the affected SC cupula and move the free-floating debris [1–3,7]. Several maneuvers have been proposed to properly diagnose each BPPV variant by moving the patient's head along the plane of the examined SC [1–3]. The "minimum stimulus strategy" represents a nystagmus-based approach aimed at minimizing the patient's discomfort, reducing the amount of diagnostic and therapeutic maneuvers required for BPPV diagnosis and treatment [8,9].

BPPV can be effectively managed by repositioning maneuvers, namely non-invasive procedures meant to move back displaced debris towards the utriculus. The canalith repositioning procedure (CRP) proposed by Epley is the most commonly used technique for the treatment of BPPV involving the PSC, which represents the most common subtype of BPPV [1,3].

Following successful repositioning maneuvers for BPPV, patients often experience light-headedness, short-lasting unsteadiness, or a persistent non-positional imbalance of variable duration. These residual symptoms, also called residual dizziness (RD), more frequently occur in older patients and in subjects with anxiety-related disorders [10–13]. Several hypotheses have been proposed to explain the pathomechanism underlying residual symptoms after successful repositioning procedures. Possible explanations include either the persistence within the canal lumen of a too limited number of residual debris to provoke detectable positional nystagmus, the persistence of utricular dysfunction accompanying BPPV, and the occurrence of long-lasting central adaptation mechanisms [14–21]. In previous research, the overall prevalence of RD ranges between 36.6% and 61% [10], and both vestibular rehabilitation and various drugs have been proposed to manage this condition [22–24].

This study evaluates the relationship between the resumption of regular daily physical and the development of RD after the successful treatment of PSC-BPPV.

2. Materials and Methods

In this prospective observational trial, we enrolled 76 patients (30 male and 46 female) admitted to the emergency room for vertigo who were diagnosed with PSC-BPPV.

Patients affected by other BPPV forms, multiple semicircular canals involvement or with a history consistent with previous vestibular disorders other than BPPV were excluded, as were patients who missed the scheduled follow-up visits. Subjects with simultaneous temporary physical impediments associated with BPPV (for example, traumatic pathologies reducing the ability to move) were also excluded.

All the patients received a bedside neurotological evaluation, including an examination of ocular alignment, saccades, smooth pursuit, and gait. Both spontaneous and gaze-evoked nystagmus with and without fixation were checked using infrared video-Frenzel goggles. According to our nystagmus-based approach, the patients underwent diagnostic positioning tests for BPPV according to the minimum stimulus strategy [25,26]. PSC-BPPV was diagnosed if the Dix–Hallpike test evoked typical paroxysmal nystagmus (up-beating and torsional nystagmus with the upper pole of the eyes beating toward the undermost ear, lasting < 1 min).

If the positional tests were consistent with PSC-BPPV, CRP, as described by Epley [3], was immediately performed. No drug was prescribed before or after physical therapy. A Dix–Hallpike maneuver was repeated about 5 min after the treatment and CRP was defined as "successful" if positional nystagmus was no longer detectable and the patient did not complain of vertigo at the control diagnostic test. Otherwise, the first CRP was defined as "ineffective" and repeated up to three times, checking the treatment result following each maneuver. In cases of ineffective CRP, the patients were re-evaluated after three days with the same protocol. A maximum of two sessions (six CRP) per patient was carried out. Patients were excluded from the study if more than two sessions were required or a canal switch occurred.

Three days after successful CRP, each patient underwent a telephone interview consisting of three dichotomous questions, to which the only possible answers were "YES" or "NO". The first question, aimed to identify the persistence of dizziness during rotational and flexion-extension head movements, was: "Do you still feel dizzy when moving your head, lying down, turning in bed and getting up from supine?". In case the answer was "YES" (persistence of positional symptoms), the interview concluded, the patient was classified as "relapses" and was invited to return to our clinic for a further check-up. Conversely, two more questions were asked if the answer was "NO" (receding of positional symptoms). The second question, aimed to verify the onset of RD, was: "Do you currently feel unsteady as you were not before the onset of BPPV?". Patients who answered "YES" were considered to have RD. Finally, the patients were asked about the resumption of their regular dynamic daily activities (RDDA) after physical therapy through the third question: "After the last successful maneuver, have you resumed the daily physical activities you were performing before the onset of BPPV?". RDDA were defined as any physical activity that patients conducted before the onset of BPPV, considering differences related to age, habits, and performance status: playing sports, swimming, jogging, cycling, walking, climbing stairs, and performing housework.

The study design is presented in Figure 1.

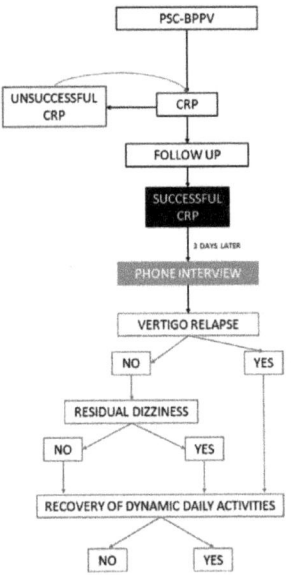

Figure 1. Study design. BPPV, benign paroxysmal positional vertigo; CRP, canalith repositioning procedure; PSC-BPPV, posterior semicircular canal BPPV.

Statistical Analysis

The continuously distributed variables were reported as mean +/− SD, after checking for normal distribution, and compared by the Student's *t*-test. The frequencies and percentages were calculated for the categorical variables, and the chi-square test was used for the comparisons.

A multivariable logistic regression model with backward stepwise variable selection was constructed to assess which factors were independently associated with the lack of RD among those highlighted in the univariate setting (sex, age, affected side, number of CRP performed, resumption of daily activities). Any p-value < 0.05 was considered statistically significant.

3. Results

Among the overall cohort of patients enrolled in the trial (n. 71), seven subjects were later excluded since five (7.04%) failed to attend the follow-up visits, while two (2.81%) required more than six CRPs.

Sixty-nine subjects were eventually included in the statistical analysis: 30 males (43.47%, mean age: 58.8 ± 13.80) and 39 females (53.13%, mean age: 57.02 ± 16.08). The affected ear was the right ear in 44 cases (63.76%). In total 39 patients (56.52%) required a single CRP to recover from PSC-BPPV, 14 (20.28%) received two CRPs, 11 (15.94%) required three CRPs, while 5 subjects received up to 6 CRPs (7.24%). The demographic data are summarized in Table 1.

Table 1. Demographic Data. DDA: Recovery of dynamic daily activities; SD: standard deviation; R: Right; L: Left; R.VERT: Relapse of vertigo; CRP: Canalith repositioning procedure; RD+: Residual dizziness development.

DDA	Subjects		Age (Mean ± SD)	Side		R. VERT	Number of CRP				RD+	RD−
				R	L		1	2	3	>4		
Yes	Male	22	58.81 ±12.90	16	6	-	11	8	2	1	4	18
	Female	27	56.70 ±18.10	16	11	3	19	3	3	2	5	19
No	Male	8	58.75 ±17.04	5	3	-	4	1	3	-	5	3
	Female	12	57.50 ±10.87	7	5	2	5	2	3	2	7	3
Tot.		69	57.79 ±15.05	44	25	5	39	14	11	5	21	43

At the telephone interview, five patients (7.24%) reported relapse of vertigo and among them, only three reported a prompt recovery of RDDA after the treatment. No differences were found in relapse occurrence according to age, sex, affected side, and number of CRPs.

Among the remaining 64 patients, 21 (32.81%) complained of RD. The statistical analysis did not show differences in RD incidence according to sex, affected side, or number of CRP. By contrast, a significant difference in the incidence of RD was found considering age: the patients who experienced RD were significantly older than those without RD (64.24 ± 12.67 vs. 53.98 ± 14.82, $p < 0.005$) (Figure 2). Among the non-relapsed patients (n. 64), 46 (71.88%) reported a complete resumption of RDDA after treatment, and 9 (19.57%) complained of RD. Conversely, among the remaining 18 patients who denied having resumed their daily activities, 12 subjects (66.67%) developed RD ($p = 0.0003$) (Figure 3).

The multivariable logistic regression model showed that patients who promptly recovered RDDA were 14 times less likely to experience RD, irrespective of sex, age, and number of CRP (OR: 14.01, 95% CI 3.14–62.47; $p = 0.001$).

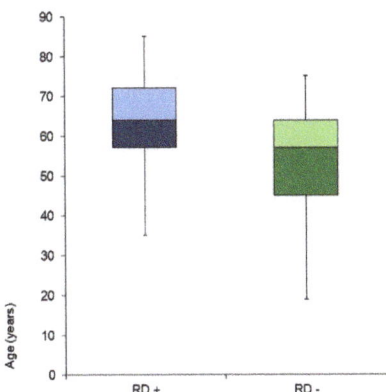

Figure 2. Residual dizziness reporting according to age. RD+, patients reporting residual dizziness; RD−, patients free from residual dizziness.

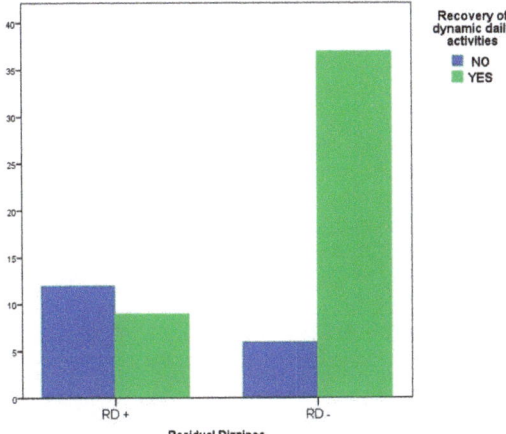

Figure 3. Correlation between residual dizziness and recovery of dynamic daily activities. RD+, patients reporting residual dizziness; RD−, patients free from residual dizziness.

4. Discussion

RD is an ambiguous disorder occurring after the successful treatment of BPPV, once positional vertigo has receded. Patients often struggle to report RD, since the disorder includes a broad spectrum of symptoms, such as a vague sense of dizziness, imbalance, light-headedness, or other balance disorders without vertigo [12].

RD is considered a complex vestibular disorder and several hypotheses have been proposed to explain its pathophysiology [14–21]. Although theoretically valid, none of them has been supported by definitive data, nor do they exclude other causal factors that could play a role in the genesis of RD acting either independently or synergistically.

Some authors assume that residual symptoms could represent a subclinical variant of BPPV due to the persistence of debris in the semicircular canal lumen. The residual otoconial matter, they argue, results in mild dizziness, although it does not provoke positional nystagmus or vertigo [18,27].

Other hypotheses focus on the role of a possible dysfunction in the utricular macula, in association with or due to BPPV. This condition could be defined as "maculo-canalopathy"; therefore, physical therapy can solve the canal dysfunction via debris removal without restoring macular function [1–3]. In support of this theory, Von Brevern et al. assessed the otolith-ocular reflex (OOR), suggesting that idiopathic BPPV is associated with utricular dysfunction and assumed that this condition could result in long-lasting imbalance after the resolution of canalolithiasis [28]. This supposition was later supported by other studies [17,29]. Furthermore, macular dysfunction due to traumatic or degenerative otoconial loss have recently been proposed as causative factors for RD [20,21].

Faralli et al. suggested that the genesis of RD could be related to the inability of the vestibular system to readjust to a new functional status quickly [16]. According to this theory, otoconial debris within the semicircular canals alter the tonic discharge of the affected labyrinth during BPPV, thereby inducing a central adaptation to rebalance the activity of vestibular nuclei, reducing peripheral asymmetry. The sudden resolution of BPPV by physical therapy alters the "new equilibrium" achieved. Therefore, central adaptation cannot promptly restore the pre-existing condition and produces subtle symptoms consistent with RD. The delayed central adaptation is associated with many factors, such as BPPV duration [10,11], age [10–16], and the subject's emotional state [12–14]. Furthermore, it should be considered that aging significantly degrades sensory systems, worsening central processes measuring balance and body perception, therefore predisposing to dizziness and disequilibrium [30]. It is well known how advancing age could increase the incidence of RD, representing an important variable to be considered [13,15]. These data are in accordance with the results of this study and with data already collected in our previous investigation [12], in which we described how age influenced the occurrence of imbalance after successful CRP. Since many factors can affect the risk of RD development, this trial included only patients with canalolithiasis affecting the posterior semicircular canal to eliminate confounding aspects related to therapeutic procedures other than CRP and misdiagnosis (i.e., central vertigo or cupulopathies mimicking BPPV). Furthermore, previous research about this topic showed that diagnostic delay is linked with a higher probability of developing RD. Therefore, only patients with recent-onset BPPV were enrolled in this trial, in order to limit the confounding factors and make the analyzed cohort more homogeneous. The presence of anxiety-related disorders, a relevant aspect in the development of residual symptoms after the resolution of BPPV, was not investigated in this earlier study.

This study mainly investigated the association between RDDA and RD. We considered the resumption of RDDA as a purely qualitative and subjective parameter, which was assessed by asking patients whether they resumed the motor activities they usually performed before the first vertigo spell after successful CRP. Each subject follows a daily routine involving repeated motor activities, regardless of age and habits. This routine varies from case to case: naturally, the RDDA of a young and fitness-focused patient will be different from that of an elderly subject with a sedentary lifestyle. However, considering our population's differences according to age and habits, attempting to quantify each patient's physical activity before and after BPPV would have been complicated and probably not very accurate. A solid association between RDDA resumption and the absence of RD, regardless of the subjects' age, was found. The data obtained from our analysis can be interpreted in two ways: the RDDA may prevent RD but, conversely, RD could prevent the resumption of the RDDA. The first hypothesis aligns with the different proposed pathogenetic theories underlying RD.

The results obtained from our analysis are in line with the different proposed pathogenetic theories underlying RD. For example, after successful repositioning maneuvers, the head movements associated with daily motor activities might be able to disperse the residual otoconial fragments in the canal lumen, preventing further perturbations on the cupula.

Although RD is mostly a self-limiting condition, patients can sometimes develop enough discomfort and disabling symptoms to require physical treatment and vestibular rehabilitation, in combination with medications if needed [31].

Drugs play an unclear role in the management of patients suffering from RD. Several medications have been proposed to approach RD, but nothing has yet been proven to provide relief for this disorder compared to placebo [13]. Albeit with conflicting results, the most commonly used molecule to approach RD is betahistine [22,24,31]. According to a randomized controlled trial, dimenhydrinate is a vestibular suppressant that could help prevent RD. However, it presents some side effects, limiting its use by selected patients for a limited number of days [32]. A prospective multicentric study reported the beneficial effect of supplementation with a polyphenol compound [23].

Vestibular rehabilitation has been developed to treat patients with chronic vestibular symptoms through a tailored exercise-based program. Vestibular rehabilitation, thanks to the development of vestibular habituation, adaptation, and substitution to enhance gaze and postural stability, is proven to improve daily functional performance [31,33].

Rodrigues et al. demonstrated that vestibular exercises in association with CRP could increase the benefit of treatments for patients with BPPV, resulting a reduction in residual symptoms and a decreasing recurrence rate [34]. Therefore, considering RD as the effect of either macular imbalance or delayed central compensation, RDDA would ideally act similarly to vestibular rehabilitation, readjusting the affected utricular function, although without the proper structure and goals. Assuming that the daily activities that are usually performed consist of systematic repetitions of space-oriented movements, it could be hypothesized that the resumption of RDDA could act centrally, rebalancing the peripheral asymmetry that occurs while otoconia are free to move within the semicircular canal. However, considering the hypothesis of permanent utricular dysfunction, the role of RDDA in preventing RD appears justified, since it might enhance neuroplasticity phenomena, making the vestibular system more receptive to natural compensatory mechanisms [34].

Nevertheless, some authors have associated the resumption of physical activity after physical therapy with BPPV relapse. For this reason, postural restrictions in the first days following physical therapy have been proposed, although this practice appears to be unjustified based on current evidence [35,36]. In our series, no differences were found in BPPV relapse subsequent to RDDA, according to previous studies.

The present study features some limitations. Firstly, it involved only patients recruited in the emergency room, with recent-onset BPPV. Since the occurrence of RD is positively related with the duration of BPPV [10,11], we could not establish whether RDDA would have played the same role in a cohort of patients with long-lasting BPPV. Furthermore, the vestibular function was not investigated instrumentally after physical therapy nor, at the follow-up evaluation. Thus, we could not analyze the effects of RDDA in case of hypothetical utricular damage.

5. Conclusions

The prompt resumption of RDDA is associated with a lack of RD after physical therapy in patients admitted to the emergency room with BPPV, regardless of age and without increasing the risk of relapses.

Author Contributions: S.M., drafting of the article, revision of the article, final approval; A.S., data collection, drafting of the article, revision of the article, final approval; A.C., statistical analysis, revision of the article, final approval; G.P., study proposal, revision of the article, final approval; V.C., data collection, analysis, final approval; V.T., statistical analysis, revision of the article, final approval; P.M., analysis, drafting of the article, final approval; G.A., analysis, data collection, final approval; F.G., analysis, data collection, final approval; A.G., study proposal, revision of the article, final approval. All authors have read and agreed to the published version of the manuscript.

Funding: This research received no external funding.

Institutional Review Board Statement: This study was approved by our Institutional Review Boards (approval number for the promoter center:126.2, Lazio-2 Ethics Committee).

Informed Consent Statement: Informed consent was obtained from all subjects involved in the study.

Data Availability Statement: The data presented in this study are available on request from the corresponding author. The data are not publicly available due to the privacy.

Conflicts of Interest: The authors received no specific funding for this research and have no financial conflict of interest.

References

1. von Brevern, M.; Bertholon, P.; Brandt, T.; Fife, T.; Imai, T.; Nuti, D.; Newman-Toker, D. Benign paroxysmal positional vertigo: Diagnostic criteria. *J. Vestib. Res.* **2015**, *25*, 105–117. [CrossRef] [PubMed]
2. Nuti, D.; Zee, D.S.; Mandalà, M. Benign Paroxysmal Positional Vertigo: What We Do and Do Not Know. *Semin. Neurol.* **2020**, *40*, 49–58. [CrossRef] [PubMed]
3. Bhattacharyya, N.; Gubbels, S.P.; Schwartz, S.R.; Edlow, J.A.; El-Kashlan, H.; Fife, T.; Holmberg, J.M.; Mahoney, K.; Hollingsworth, D.B.; Roberts, R.; et al. Clinical Practice Guideline: Benign paroxysmal positional vertigo (update). *Otolaryngol. Neck Surg.* **2017**, *156*, S1–S47. [CrossRef]
4. Castellucci, A.; Malara, P.; Martellucci, S.; Botti, C.; Delmonte, S.; Quaglieri, S.; Rebecchi, E.; Armato, E.; Ralli, M.; Manfrin, M.L.; et al. Feasibility of Using the Video-Head Impulse Test to Detect the Involved Canal in Benign Paroxysmal Positional Vertigo Presenting with Positional Downbeat Nystagmus. *Front. Neurol.* **2020**, *11*, 578588. [CrossRef] [PubMed]
5. Martellucci, S.; Castellucci, A.; Malara, P.; Pagliuca, G.; Clemenzi, V.; Stolfa, A.; Gallo, A.; Libonati, G.A. Spontaneous Jamming of Horizontal Semicircular Canal Combined with Canalolithiasis of Contralateral Posterior Semicircular Canal. *J. Audiol. Otol.* **2021**, *15*. [CrossRef]
6. Castellucci, A.; Botti, C.; Martellucci, S.; Malara, P.; Delmonte, S.; Lusetti, F.; Ghidini, A. Spontaneous Upbeat Nystagmus and Selective Anterior Semicircular Canal Hypofunction on Video Head Impulse Test: A New Variant of Canalith Jam? *J. Audiol. Otol.* **2021**. [CrossRef]
7. Castellucci, A.; Malara, P.; Martellucci, S.; Delmonte, S.; Ghidini, A. Fluctuating Posterior Canal Function in Benign Paroxysmal Positional Vertigo Depending on How and Where Otoconia Are Disposed. *Otol. Neurotol.* **2021**, *42*, e193–e198. [CrossRef] [PubMed]
8. Libonati, G.A. Benign Paroxysmal Positional Vertigo and Positional Vertigo Variants. *Int. J. Otorhinolaryngol. Clin.* **2012**, *4*, 25–40. [CrossRef]
9. Malara, P.; Castellucci, A.; Martellucci, S. Upright head roll test: A new contribution for the diagnosis of lateral semicircular canal benign paroxysmal positional vertigo. *Audiol. Res.* **2020**, *10*, 236. [CrossRef]
10. Seok, J.I.; Lee, H.M.; Yoo, J.H.; Lee, D.K. Residual dizziness after successful repositioning treatment in patients with benign paroxysmal positional vertigo. *J. Clin. Neurol.* **2008**, *4*, 107–110. [CrossRef] [PubMed]
11. Teggi, R.; Giordano, L.; Bondi, S.; Fabiano, B.; Bussi, M. Residual dizziness after successful repositioning maneuvers for idiopathic benign paroxysmal positional vertigo in the elderly. *Eur. Arch. Oto-Rhino-Laryngol.* **2010**, *268*, 507–511. [CrossRef]
12. Martellucci, S.; Pagliuca, G.; de Vincentiis, M.; Greco, A.; De Virgilio, A.; Benedetti, F.M.N.; Gallipoli, C.; Rosato, C.; Clemenzi, V.; Gallo, A. Features of Residual Dizziness after Canalith Repositioning Procedures for Benign Paroxysmal Positional Vertigo. *Otolaryngol. Neck Surg.* **2016**, *154*, 693–701. [CrossRef]
13. Giommetti, G.; Lapenna, R.; Panichi, R.; Mobaraki, P.D.; Longari, F.; Ricci, G.; Faralli, M. Residual Dizziness after Successful Repositioning Maneuver for Idiopathic Benign Paroxysmal Positional Vertigo: A Review. *Audiol. Res.* **2017**, *7*, 178. [CrossRef]
14. Faralli, M.; Ricci, G.; Ibba, M.C.; Crognoletti, M.; Longari, F.; Frenguelli, A. Dizziness in patients with recent episodes of benign paroxysmal positional vertigo: Real otolithic dysfunction or mental stress? *J. Otolaryngol.-Head Neck Surg.* **2009**, *38*, 375–380.
15. Wu, P.; Yang, J.; Huang, X.; Ma, Z.; Zhang, T.; Li, H. Predictors of residual dizziness in patients with benign paroxysmal positional vertigo after successful repositioning: A multi-center prospective cohort study. *J. Vestib. Res.* **2021**, *31*, 119–129. [CrossRef] [PubMed]
16. Faralli, M.; Lapenna, R.; Giommetti, G.; Pellegrino, C.; Ricci, G. Residual dizziness after the first BPPV episode: Role of otolithic function and of a delayed diagnosis. *Eur. Arch. Oto-Rhino-Laryngol.* **2016**, *273*, 3157–3165. [CrossRef] [PubMed]
17. Seo, T.; Shiraishi, K.; Kobayashi, T.; Mutsukazu, K.; Fujita, T.; Saito, K.; Watanabe, H.; Doi, K. Residual dizziness after successful treatment of idiopathic benign paroxysmal positional vertigo originates from persistent utricular dysfunction. *Acta Oto-Laryngol.* **2017**, *137*, 1149–1152. [CrossRef] [PubMed]
18. Dispenza, F.; Mazzucco, W.; Mazzola, S.; Martines, F. Observational study on risk factors determining residual dizziness after successful benign paroxysmal positional vertigo treatment: The role of subclinical BPPV. *Acta Otorhinolaryngol. Ital.* **2019**, *39*, 347–352. [CrossRef]
19. Martellucci, S.; Attanasio, G.; Ralli, M.; Marcelli, V.; de Vincentiis, M.; Greco, A.; Gallo, A. Does cervical range of motion affect the outcomes of canalith repositioning procedures for posterior canal benign positional paroxysmal vertigo? *Am. J. Otolaryngol.* **2019**, *40*, 494–498. [CrossRef]
20. Suh, K.D.; Oh, S.R.; Chae, H.; Lee, S.Y.; Chang, M.; Mun, S.-K. Can Osteopenia Induce Residual Dizziness After Treatment of Benign Paroxysmal Positional Vertigo? *Otol. Neurotol.* **2020**, *41*, e603–e606. [CrossRef]
21. Hegemann, S.C.A.; Weisstanner, C.; Ernst, A.; Basta, D.; Bockisch, C.J. Constant severe imbalance following traumatic otoconial loss: A new explanation of residual dizziness. *Eur. Arch. Oto-Rhino-Laryngol.* **2020**, *277*, 2427–2435. [CrossRef]
22. Jalali, M.M.; Gerami, H.; Saberi, A.; Razaghi, S. The Impact of Betahistine versus Dimenhydrinate in the Resolution of Residual Dizziness in Patients with Benign Paroxysmal Positional Vertigo: A Randomized Clinical Trial. *Ann. Otol. Rhinol. Laryngol.* **2020**, *129*, 434–440. [CrossRef]
23. Casani, A.P.; Navari, E.; Albera, R.; Agus, G.; Libonati, G.A.; Chiarella, G.; Lombardo, N.; Marcelli, V.; Ralli, G.; di Santillo, L.S.; et al. Approach to residual dizziness after successfully treated benign paroxysmal positional vertigo: Effect of a polyphenol compound supplementation. *Clin. Pharmacol.* **2019**, *11*, 117–125. [CrossRef]

24. Acar, B.; Karasen, R.M.; Buran, Y. Efficacy of medical therapy in the prevention of residual dizziness after successful repositioning maneuvers for Benign Paroxysmal Positional Vertigo (BPPV). *B-ENT* **2015**, *11*, 117–121. [PubMed]
25. Libonati, G.A. Diagnostic and treatment strategy of lateral semicircular canal canalolithiasis. *Acta Otorhinolaryngol. Ital.* **2005**, *25*, 277–283.
26. Martellucci, S.; Malara, P.; Castellucci, A.; Pecci, R.; Giannoni, B.; Marcelli, V.; Scarpa, A.; Cassandro, E.; Quaglieri, S.; Manfrin, M.L.; et al. Upright BPPV Protocol: Feasibility of a New Diagnostic Paradigm for Lateral Semicircular Canal Benign Paroxysmal Positional Vertigo Compared to Standard Diagnostic Maneuvers. *Front. Neurol.* **2020**, *11*. [CrossRef]
27. Di Girolamo, S.; Paludetti, G.; Briglia, G.; Cosenza, A.; Santarelli, R.; Di Nardo, W. Postural control in benign paroxysmal positional vertigo before and after recovery. *Acta Otolaryngol.* **1998**, *118*, 289–293.
28. Von Brevern, M.; Schmidt, T.; Schönfeld, U.; Lempert, T.; Clarke, A.H. Utricular dysfunction in patients with benign paroxysmal positional vertigo. *Otol. Neurotol.* **2006**, *27*, 92–96. [CrossRef]
29. Yetiser, S.; Ince, D.; Gül, M. An Analysis of Vestibular Evoked Myogenic Potentials in patients with benign paroxysmal positional vertigo. *Ann. Otol. Rhinol. Laryngol.* **2014**, *123*, 686–695. [CrossRef] [PubMed]
30. D'Elia, A.; Quaranta, N.; Libonati, G.A.; Ralli, G.; Morelli, A.; Inchingolo, F.; Cialdella, F.; Martellucci, S.; Barbara, F. The cochleo-vestibular secretory senescence. *J. Gerontol. Geriatr.* **2020**, *68*, 85–90. [CrossRef]
31. Wu, P.; Cao, W.; Hu, Y.; Li, H. Effects of vestibular rehabilitation, with or without betahistine, on managing residual dizziness after successful repositioning manoeuvres in patients with benign paroxysmal positional vertigo: A protocol for a randomized controlled trial. *BMJ Open* **2019**, *9*, e026711. [CrossRef] [PubMed]
32. Kim, M.-B.; Lee, H.S.; Ban, J.H. Vestibular suppressants after canalith repositioning in benign paroxysmal positional vertigo. *Laryngoscope* **2014**, *124*, 2400–2403. [CrossRef] [PubMed]
33. Han, B.I.; Song, H.S.; Kim, J.S. Vestibular rehabilitation therapy: Review of indications, mechanisms, and key exercises. *J. Clin. Neurol.* **2011**, *7*, 184–196. [CrossRef] [PubMed]
34. Rodrigues, D.L.; Ledesma, A.L.L.; de Oliveira, C.A.P.; Bahmad, F. Effect of vestibular exercises associated with repositioning maneuvers in patients with benign paroxysmal positional vertigo: A randomized controlled clinical trial. *Otol. Neurotol.* **2019**, *40*, e824–e829. [CrossRef] [PubMed]
35. Marciano, E.; Marcelli, V. Postural restrictions in labyrintholithiasis. *Eur. Arch. Oto-Rhino-Laryngol.* **2002**, *259*, 262–265. [CrossRef] [PubMed]
36. Fyrmpas, G.; Rachovitsas, D.; Haidich, A.B.; Constantinidis, J.; Triaridis, S.; Vital, V.; Tsalighopoulos, M. Are postural restrictions after an Epley maneuver unnecessary? First results of a controlled study and review of the literature. *Auris Nasus Larynx* **2009**, *36*, 637–643. [CrossRef]

Article

Sulcus Vocalis and Benign Vocal Cord Lesions: Is There Any Relationship?

Carmelo Saraniti , Gaetano Patti and Barbara Verro *

Division of Otorhinolaryngology, Department of Biomedicine, Neuroscience and Advanced Diagnostic, University of Palermo, 90127 Palermo, Italy
* Correspondence: verrobarbara@gmail.com

Abstract: Background: Sulcus vocalis (SV) is a longitudinal groove in the free edge of the true vocal cord. It may impair phonation with incomplete glottic closure, phonasthenia and hoarseness. This study aims to detect a correlation between benign vocal cord lesions and the incidence of the SV. Methods: A retrospective study was carried out on patients who underwent transoral surgery due to benign vocal fold lesions and were selected according to strict criteria. Patients were divided into a group with sulcus vocalis (Group wSV) and a group without sulcus vocalis (Group w/oSV). The possible correlations between variables were assessed by the Pearson chi-square test ($p < 0.05$). Results: The study included 232 vocal cord lesions in 229 patients: 62.88% were females whose mean age was 46.61 ± 14.04. The most frequent diseases were polyps (37.94%), nodules (18.53%) and Reinke's edema (21.12%). Statistically significant relationships were found between age and SV (p-value 0.0005) and between mild dysplasia and SV (p-value 0.03). Conclusions: This study did not detect a cause–effect relationship between SV and benign vocal fold lesions. SV within vocal fold lesions is more common in younger patients, suggesting a congenital nature of SV. In conclusion, in the case of a benign vocal fold lesion, a possible SV should be considered and researched to provide the patient the best healthcare.

Keywords: larynx; laryngoscopic surgery; phonation; voice quality; vocal cords

1. Introduction

The vocal fold is composed of squamous epithelium, lamina propria (superficial, intermediate and deep layers) and vocal muscle. Vocal fold lesions may lead to dysfunction due to the loss of elasticity and integrity of the vocal fold [1]. Sulcus vocalis (SV) is a longitudinal groove in the free edge of the true vocal cord; it represents an area of decreased mucosal elasticity. Indeed, this lesion changes the normal physiology of the vocal folds with impaired glottic closure, vocal fatigue, phonasthenia and hoarseness [2–4]. Typical dysphonia is characterized by a high-pitched and diplophonic breathy voice. Sulcus vocalis was first reported by anatomist Giacomini in 1892, who described it as an abnormality in the vocal cord [5]. Ford et al. [6] classified this lesion in three degrees of severity: type I with no functional effect and called physiological sulcus; type II, or sulcus vergeture, with a loss of the superficial layer of lamina propria; and type III, which Selleck et al. [7] consider the true sulcus vocalis, with a mucosal-loss focal area in the vocal ligament or deeper (also called pocket-type). The last two types of sulcus vocalis are considered pathological sulcus. Making the diagnosis of sulcus vocalis can be challenging. In fact, the incidence of SV is not clear and ranges from 0.4% to 48% according to various articles [3,4]. The patient should be examined by an ENT and a speech therapist to give a global approach to the disease. In fact, the vocal cords may appear normal during in-office laryngoscopy, whereas videostroboscopy can easily highlight a vocal cord lesion. Hirano et al. described usual findings during laryngoscopy: bow-shaped vocal cords with incomplete glottic closure (the so-called "spindle-shaped pattern") and medial invaginations (almost splitting the vocal fold), a reduced mucosal wave and supraglottic hyperactivity as a compensatory mechanism [8]. However, these features can also be found in vocal cord atrophy; thus, it is important to detect the sulcus to make a differential diagnosis. In their studies, Dailey et al. and Akbulut et al. [9,10] also reported difficulties in making diagnoses of sulcus vocalis using videostroboscopy. Indeed, in cases of moderate to severe dysphonia, videostroboscopy cannot provide clear and accurate information due to failed synchronization (the fundamental frequency F0 cannot be recorded). Moreover, this exam provides qualitative data, resulting in high inter-individual variability [11]. Dailey et al. stated that SV is the most undiagnosed benign vocal cord lesion in patients examined due to benign glottic disease [9]. These drawbacks make it difficult to elaborate precise statistical studies since the diagnostic evaluation is operator-dependent. Indeed, in-office laryngoscopy provides a view tangent to SV and vocal fold lesions, resulting in difficulty to detect the sulcus itself (the authors called it the "umbrella effect") [12].

Several therapeutic strategies, surgical and non-surgical, can be chosen since today there is no consensus about the best therapy. Voice therapy can be accepted in the first instance [13,14]; however, when the speech-therapy treatment is ineffective and functional limitations and worse quality of voice occur, a surgical treatment can be proposed: medialization laryngoplasty [15,16], pulsed laser treatment [17,18], vocal fold injections [19–21] or autologous tissue implantation [22–33]. To date, the latter seems to be the best therapeutic choice for the success of vocal cord flexibility and for long-term outcomes. Indeed, treatment of SV should achieve two goals: restoring the mucosal wave and fixing the anatomic abnormality.

Furthermore, sulcus vocalis seems to be correlated with coexisting vocal cord lesions. As reported in a few reviews [24–27], in cases of benign vocal fold lesions, a sulcus vocalis should always be considered since treating the benign lesion but leaving out the sulcus may not lead to the complete improvement of the patient's symptoms, in addition to causing a predisposition to phonotrauma.

Based on these premises and on the poor literature, this study aims to evaluate the incidence of sulcus vocalis in patients undergoing transoral laryngeal surgery (TOLS) due to vocal cord pathology, seeking a correlation between the presence of a sulcus and the onset of benign vocal cord lesions.

2. Materials and Methods

2.1. Study Design

A retrospective study was carried out on patients who underwent TOLS due to benign vocal fold lesions from January 2010 to January 2020 in our Ear Nose and Throat Clinic at the University Hospital of Palermo. This study was approved by the ethical committee of our university hospital (approval number: 04/2022), and informed consent was obtained from the patients in accordance with the Helsinki Declaration.

The inclusion criteria were as follows: males and females aged between 18 and 80 years old, patients undergoing TOLS due to vocal cord lesions and histological diagnosis of a benign vocal fold lesion.

The exclusion criteria were as follows: histological diagnosis of malignant vocal fold lesions (severe dysplasia, carcinoma in situ or carcinoma) and patients undergoing TOLS due to non-vocal cord lesions.

The following data were collected: demography (age and sex), surgical technique (cold or laser surgery), histological diagnosis (nodules, polyps, Reinke's edema, cyst, papillomatosis or others), side (right and/or left vocal cord) and number of vocal cord lesions (mono or bilateral) and presence or not and side of sulcus. Recruited patients were divided into two groups: a group of patients with sulcus vocalis (Group wSV) and a group of patients without sulcus vocalis (Group w/oSV).

2.2. Data Analysis

Data on the demography, surgery, vocal fold lesion and sulci of the recruited patients were collected in a data spreadsheet using Microsoft Excel, version 16.66.1. These data were reported as numbers and percentages of the total and/or mean ± standard deviation (SD). MedCalc software was used for the statistical analyses. The possible associations between the dichotomous nominal variables were assessed by calculating the Pearson chi-square tests [34]. A *p*-value of <0.05 was considered statistically significant.

3. Results

The study included 232 vocal cord lesions in 229 patients: 144 (62.88%) females and 85 (37.12%) males aged between 18 and 80 years old (the mean age was 46.61 ± 14.04). In particular, 77 (33.62%) patients belonged to Group wSV, and 152 (66.38%) belonged to Group w/oSV.

All patients were treated by the same surgeon (CS) to avoid biases related to different surgeons' skills. Moreover, due to the difficulty in detecting a sulcus during an in-office laryngoscopy, we included in this study only cases where a sulcus was confirmed during the surgical procedure.

Vocal fold lesions included in the analysis were: angioma (0.43%), polyp (37.94%), nodule (18.53%), cyst (9.05%), papillomatosis (0.86%), Reinke's edema (21.12%) and mild (6.03%) and moderate (3.02%) dysplasia. The data are summarized in Table 1. The most frequent diseases were polyps (37.94%), nodules (18.53%) and Reinke's edema (21.12%) (Figures 1 and 2). In particular, as regards Group wSV, polyps were the most common finding (44.30%), followed by nodules and Reinke's edema, which had the same incidence (20.25%). No cases of papillomatosis and/or moderate dysplasia were reported for this group.

Table 1. Characteristics of included patients and results of possible associations between variables.

Characteristics	Group wSV (%)	Group w/oSV (%)	Total (%)	Chi-Square (*p*-Value)
Sex				
Female	52 (67.53)	92 (60.53)	144 (62.88)	1.07 (0.299)
Male	25 (32.47)	60 (39.47)	85 (37.12)	
Age				
Mean ± SD	42.09 ± 12.00	48.90 ± 14.44	46.61 ± 14.04	14.92 (0.0005)
Range	18–74	18–80	18–80	
18–44 years old	45 (58.44)	55 (36.18)		
45–64 years old	30 (38.96)	72 (47.37)		
65–80 years old	2 (2.60)	25 (16.45)		
Angioma	1 (1.27)	0 (0)	1 (0.43)	
Left	1	0	1	-
Right	0	0	0	
Bilateral	0	0	0	
Polyp	35 (44.30)	53 (34.64)	88 (37.94)	
Left	10	13	23	2.42 (0.11)
Right	13	26	39	
Bilateral	12	14	26	
Nodule	16 (20.25)	27 (17.65)	43 (18.53)	
Left	2	5	8	0.304 (0.58)
Right	7	16	23	
Bilateral	6	6	32	

Table 1. Cont.

Characteristics	Group wSV (%)	Group w/oSV (%)	Total (%)	Chi-Square (p-Value)
Cyst	7 (8.86)	14 (9.15)	21 (9.05)	
Left	3	7	10	0.0009 (0.97)
Right	4	6	10	
Bilateral	0	1	1	
Reinke's edema	16 (20.25)	33 (21.57)	49 (21.12)	0.026 (0.87)
Papillomatosis	0 (0)	2 (1.31)	2 (0.86)	
Left	0	0	0	
Right	0	1	1	-
Bilateral	0	1	1	
Keratosis	3 (3.80)	4 (2.61)	7 (3.02)	
Left	0	2	2	0.275 (0.59)
Right	3	0	3	
Bilateral	0	2	2	
Mild dysplasia	1 (1.27)	13 (8.50)	14 (6.03)	
Left	0	1	1	4.68 (0.03)
Right	0	5	5	
Bilateral	1	7	8	
Moderate dysplasia	0 (0)	7 (4.57)	7 (3.02)	
Left	0	1	1	-
Right	0	3	3	
Bilateral	0	3	3	
Total	79 (34.05)	153 (65.95)	232 (100)	

There are 232 vocal fold lesions and 229 patients because we had 2 patients with a right nodule and a left cyst and 1 patient with a right polyp and a left nodule.

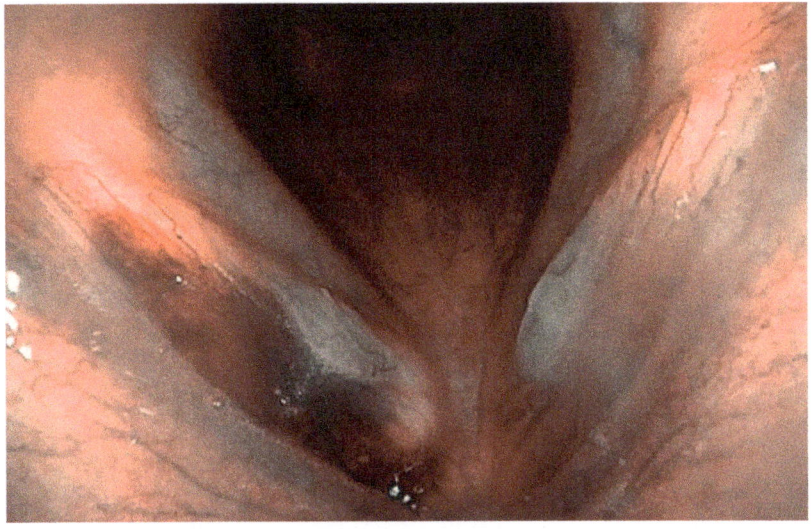

Figure 1. Bilateral sulcus with bilateral nodules and a right vocal cord hemorrhage due to phonotrauma (Narrow-Band Imaging).

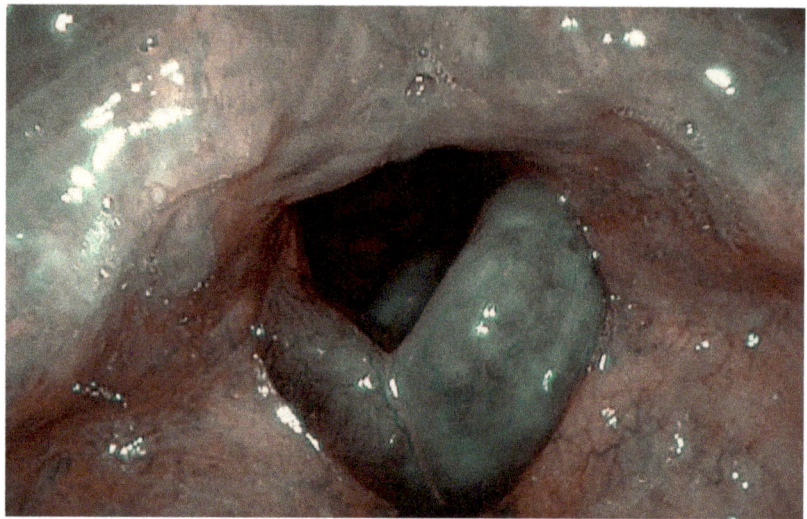

Figure 2. Bilateral sulcus in Reinke's edema (Narrow-Band Imaging).

In both groups, female prevalence was found: 67.53% for Group wSV and 60.53% for Group w/oSV. However, statistical analysis did not show any statistically significant correlation between the variable "sex" and the presence/absence of sulci (p-value 0.299).

Patients were divided into three age categories: (1) young people (18–44 years old), (2) middle-aged people (45–64 years old) and (3) older people (65–80 years old). The study revealed that most patients in Group wSV were young (58.44%), while 47.37% of the patients who belonged to Group w/oSV were aged between 45 and 64 years old. The chi-square test showed a statistically significant relationship between age and the presence of sulci (p-value 0.0005).

No association was found between the type of vocal cord lesion and the presence of a sulcus, except for mild dysplasia (p-value 0.03).

Also, a possible correlation between the side of the lesion and the side of the sulcus was evaluated by the chi-square test calculator for a 3 × 3 contingency table with a negative result (p-value 0.08) (Table 2). The SV was bilateral in 31 cases (40.26%), and 25.96% of the patients had both bilateral SV and bilateral vocal fold lesions.

Table 2. Study of the correlation between the side of the lesion and the side of the sulcus.

Sulcus side	Lesion Side			Total
	Right	Left	Bilateral	
Right	13	4	11	28
Left	5	4	9	18
Bilateral	4	7	20	31
Total	22	15	40	77
Chi-square (p-value)	8.2228 (0.08)			

4. Discussion

Sulcus vocalis is a longitudinal furrow that runs along the vocal cords, altering not only the vocal cords' anatomy but their functionality, too. Vocal fold scarring means that the mucosa is tethered to the underlying tissue and cannot vibrate freely, causing vocal fatigue, incomplete glottic closure and hoarseness [1–4,6,7,9]. As written above, the vocal folds are composed of the cover (epithelium and superficial layer of lamina propria) and body (intermediate and deep layers of lamina propria and vocal muscle). As described by Hirano in 1975, according to the cover-body theory, during phonation, the airflow from the trachea leads to the vibration of the pliable cover on the body of the vocal folds [35,36]. A study by Zhou et al. demonstrated that sulcus vocalis causes a directly proportional increase in the phonation threshold pressure. This increase requires more effort to be made to provide adequate airflow. This effort results in hoarseness, vocal fatigue, phonasthenia and worse voice quality. Obviously, the effort and symptoms worsen with increasing sulcus depth [37]. As reported by Hirano et al., the vocal fatigue and hoarseness are due more to incomplete glottic closure than to stiff vocal folds [8]. Stroboscopic studies show a statistically significant increase in the mean F0 in types II and III of sulcus vocalis [38].

In 1994, Pontes et al. suggested a first classification of sulcus vocalis into the following categories: (1) sulcus stria minor, which is an epithelial depression; (2) sulcus stria major, where the mucosal invagination adheres to the deep layer, vocal ligament and muscle; and (3) pouch-shaped sulcus lesion, where the invagination results into a pouch-shaped subepithelial depression [38]. However, the most common classification was formed by Ford et al. in 1996 [6], dividing sulcus vocalis into three categories: type I, or physiologic sulcus; type II, also called sulcus vergeture; and type III, which is the "true sulcus vocalis" or a pouch-like depression [7].

The etiology of sulcus vocalis is still unclear today. The ideas of the various authors are controversial, and the scientific literature is lacking in this regard. Bouchayer et al. [1] and Ford et al. [6] ascribe these causes to gastroesophageal reflux, laryngeal chronic inflammation, errors in surgical technique, congenital alterations, mucosal atrophies, embryonic defects and others. In particular, Bouchayer et al. assumed that sulcus vocalis is the result of the rupture of an epidermoid cyst from remnants of the fourth and sixth brachial arches. According to this theory, the capsule of the epidermoid cyst has remained attached to the deep tissues of the vocal cords, resulting in the formation of an invagination that is the sulcus [1]. Moreover, Sato et al. studied the mucosa of sulcus vocalis using electron microscopy and demonstrating degenerated and fewer fibroblasts in the macula flava, resulting in changes in elastic and collagenous fibers in the vocal fold mucosa [39]. Lee et al. analyzed the histology of surgical specimens and found epithelial changes (parakeratosis, dyskeratosis and inflammatory infiltrate) in most of the cases. Based on these findings, the authors suggested a similarity with the pathogenesis of cholesteatoma [38]. Indeed, SV has a pouch-like appearance, as well as a retraction pocket of the tympanic membrane that promotes keratin accumulation and subsequent inflammation. This excessive immune response is responsible for subepithelial vocal fold damage and impaired voice quality. These epithelial changes may explain the common finding of benign vocal fold lesions with SV.

After studying four individuals of the same family with dysphonia, Martins et al. [31,32] suggested a genetic origin of sulci, such as autosomal dominant inheritance. However, the authors state that is not possible to establish a genetic transmission of this disorder.

Moreover, based on the current literature, sulcus vocalis does not seem to predominantly affect a gender or a specific age. Itoh et al. [2] studied 240 patients who were divided into three groups: (1) sulcus with hoarseness, (2) sulcus with another laryngeal disease and (3) sulcus with no vocal disorder. The study found that 72% were male and that most of the patients were aged between 60 and 69 years old. The lesions were bilateral in 63% of the patients and unilateral in 37%, with no significant difference between the right and left sides. On the contrary, Sünter et al. [27] found that 56.4% of patients with sulci and benign vocal cord lesions were female, without reporting a significance difference in gender, with a mean age of 43.50 ± 12.7. In addition, in our study, most of the patients with sulci were females (67.53%) and were young, aged between 18 and 44 years old (58.44%), with a mean age of 42.09 ± 12.00. Varelas et al. suggest that the female prevalence may be due to anatomic and physiologic features. Indeed, women have smaller and thinner vocal cords and a higher F0 than men, meaning that they have increased fold vibration and, so, a higher risk to develop voice diseases due to phonotrauma [38]. Thus, the prevalence of women with SV in studies may be related to higher incidence of benign vocal fold lesions. Moreover, we found a statistically significant correlation between age and sulcus ($p = 0.0005$). Sünter et al. suggested that the young age of occurrence could be explained by a congenital sulcus [27].

However, regarding a possible correlation between the side and number of sulci and the side and number of vocal cord lesions, we did not find any statistical difference ($p \geq 0.05$), as was reported by Itoh et al. [2]. Instead, in 2018, Carmel-Neiderman et al. [28] tried to detect a correlation between vocal fold polyps (VFP) and sulcus vocalis and found that patients with SV and VFP had a higher risk of developing contralateral vocal fold lesions due to phonotrauma ($p = 0.04$). A vocal polyp is a lesion of epithelium and a superficial layer of the lamina propria of the vocal fold; its onset is usually linked to vocal misuse and abuse due to possible pre-existing sulcus vocalis, resulting in phonotrauma. This assumption explains why the polyp usually develops on the same side as the SV.

In addition, in our study, the VFP was the most frequently found benign lesion in Group wSV (44.30%), although no statistically significant correlation was demonstrated.

Moreover, the study of Byeon et al. [31] supported our hypothesis that, in cases of the co-presence of SV and benign vocal fold lesions, the surgical treatment of the lesion without fixing the sulcus, may increase the risk of recurrence of the lesion itself. Indeed, in their study, the authors reported a significantly higher recurrence rate of VFP in the group with SV (16.7%) than in the group without SV (3.1%).

Moreover, in their casuistry, Sünter et al. [27] did not report the simultaneous presence of bilateral vocal nodules and SV. The authors explained that it is predictable since they have the same vocal fold localization, and SV usually causes phonotrauma around the sulcus itself. On the contrary, we found that 20.25% of Group wSV had vocal nodules without a statistical correlation with SV. Soares et al. stressed that most patients have bilateral sulcus vocalis (77%) [40]. The same results were observed by Yildiz et al., who found that 100% of included patients had bilateral SV [11]. In our study, we found a similar result: 40.26% of patients were affected by bilateral SV.

Nakayama et al. [33] studied sulcus vocalis in laryngeal cancer patients and demonstrated that sulci were more common in the cancer group, suggesting increased susceptibility; the chronic inflammation associated with tumors in adjacent or contralateral vocal folds might be a factor in the pathogenesis of sulcus vocalis. In our study, we excluded malignant glottic lesions because this kind of lesion could make it difficult to detect sulcus and, thus, impair statistical results as a bias.

As mentioned above, over the years, several therapeutic strategies have been proposed. In particular, there are surgical and non-surgical treatments. Voice therapy is indicated and effective in cases of type I sulci and consists of exercises to reduce vocal effort and to avoid compensatory mechanisms that may lead to vocal fold lesions. Pathological sulcus vocalis needs surgical strategies that include medialization laryngoplasty (also called type I thyroplasty) and vocal fold injections. In both cases, the main goal of the surgery is the medialization of the vocal cords to reduce the glottic incompetence. Up to now, vocal fold injections represent the best therapeutic approach with the filling of different materials: autologous fat, hyaluronic acid, steroids and/or platelet-rich plasma (PRP). Autograft fat is almost the best filler since it is inexpensive, biocompatible and easy-to-harvest. Moreover, a recent study demonstrated that vocal fold injections of PRP plus fat improve the advantages of fat, leading to faster post-operative vocal cord healing, longer lasting of the filler and softening of the cover layer. Indeed, the fat plus PRP mixture allows us to reach two goals: reduction in glottic insufficiency and reduction in vocal cord stiffness. Thus, the authors demonstrated that this type of vocal fold injections could be considered the best treatment for pathological sulcus since it allows us to achieve better vocal cord movement and vibration and a reduced glottic gap, with lasting results over time and a low risk of recurrence [41].

Tsunoda et al. [24] introduced a new technique consisting of the transplantation of autologous fascia into the vocal cords with SV. The authors formulated this technique based on the use of temporal fascia during tympanoplasty. Actually, this fascia improves vocal fold healing, and it is related to a low risk of infection and immunological reactivity. In this case, the temporal fascia is placed in a pocket, which is the Reinke's space, between the cover and the body of the vocal cord. Thus, this surgery reduces the glottic gap and improves the mucosal wave during phonation.

Bouchayer et al. [1] suggested freeing the mucosa from the deeper layers of the vocal folds to restore the body-cover structure. Moreover, they suggested fixing the flap with fibrin glue. However, this so-called "epithelium freeing technique" does not allow us to overcome the glottic insufficiency, so this surgery should be associated with vocal fold injections.

However, this work has a few limits: first, it is a retrospective study, so it has less confidence and a lower level of evidence than prospective ones. In addition, we collected data from only one experienced surgeon; this could be a limit for data analysis, but this choice allowed us to avoid biases related to subjective operators' skills. Indeed, as reported by Sünter et al. [26], the diagnosis of a sulcus is sometimes only made during a direct laryngoscopy with an experienced surgeon. In this regard, a recent study suggested the use of Narrow-Band Imaging (NBI) endoscopy to better detect SV in outpatients [42], as also shown in Figures 1 and 2. Desuter et al. observed that, in cases of SV, the vessels that usually are parallel to vocal fold change their course and split, skirting the edges of the furrow. The authors called it "the lake road sign", as well as the roads that surround lakes [43]. If this finding was the rule, NBI would be useful for SV diagnosis. Lim et al. reported capillary ectasis in 35% of patients with pathologic sulci, too, as a sign of severe inflammation [44]. In 1996, Ford et al. [6] found that mucosal vessels had a perpendicular course to the vocal folds in SV, suggesting that they may be considered "herald vessels" of pathologic sulci.

5. Conclusions

Sulcus vocalis is a longitudinal, full-thickness depression in the free edge of the true vocal fold that may impair phonation, causing phonotrauma. This question was the basis of the study: is there any cause–effect relationship between sulcus vocalis and benign vocal fold lesions? However, this study did not find any statistically significant correlation, except in the case of mild dysplasia, which may be due to chronic phonotrauma from sulcus itself. Moreover, we found that SV within a vocal fold lesion is more common in younger patients, suggesting a congenital nature of SV.

In conclusion, the take-home message is that in cases of benign vocal fold lesions, a possible SV should be considered and researched for two reasons: first, the surgeon should notify to patient that, in treating SV, the voice might change further, and, second, if the surgeon fails to heal the SV, the risk of recurrence of vocal fold lesion would be high.

However, further studies are needed to better know SV and its role in the onset of vocal fold lesions in order to provide the patient the best healthcare.

Author Contributions: Conceptualization, C.S.; methodology, B.V.; validation, C.S. and B.V.; formal analysis, investigation and resources, G.P.; data curation, B.V.; writing—original draft preparation, B.V. and G.P.; writing—review and editing, B.V. and C.S.; supervision, C.S. All authors have read and agreed to the published version of the manuscript.

Funding: This research received no external funding.

Institutional Review Board Statement: The study was conducted in accordance with the Declaration of Helsinki and approved by the Ethics Committee Palermo 1 of University Hospital Paolo Giaccone, Palermo (protocol codes 04/2022, and 13/04/2022).

Informed Consent Statement: Informed consent was obtained from all subjects involved in the study.

Data Availability Statement: Not applicable.

Conflicts of Interest: The authors declare no conflict of interest.

References

1. Bouchayer, M.; Cornut, G.; Witzig, E.; Loire, R.; Roch, J.B.; Bastian, R.W. Epidermoid cysts, sulci, and mucosal bridges of the true vocal cord: A report of 157 cases. *Laryngoscope* **1985**, *95 Pt 1*, 1087–1094. [CrossRef] [PubMed]
2. Itoh, T.; Kawasaki, H.; Morikawa, I.; Hirano, M. Vocal fold furrows. A 10-year review of 240 patients. *Auris Nasus Larynx* **1983**, *10*, S17–S26. [CrossRef] [PubMed]
3. Xiao, Y.; Liu, F.; Ma, L.; Wang, T.; Guo, W.; Wang, J. Clinical Analysis of Benign Vocal Fold Lesions with Occult Sulcus Vocalis. *J. Voice* **2021**, *35*, 646–650. [CrossRef] [PubMed]
4. Soni, R.S.; Dailey, S.H. Sulcus Vocalis. *Otolaryngol. Clin. N. Am.* **2019**, *52*, 735–743. [CrossRef]
5. Giacomini, C. Annotazioni sull'anatomia del negro. *G. Accad. Med. Torino* **1892**, *40*, 17–61.
6. Ford, C.N.; Inagi, K.; Khidr, A.; Bless, D.M.; Gilchrist, K.W. Sulcus vocalis: A rational analytical approach to diagnosis and management. *Ann. Otol. Rhinol. Laryngol.* **1996**, *105*, 189–200. [CrossRef]
7. Selleck, A.M.; Moore, J.E.; Rutt, A.L.; Hu, A.; Sataloff, R.T. Sulcus Vocalis (Type III): Prevalence and Strobovideolaryngoscopy Characteristics. *J. Voice* **2015**, *29*, 507–511. [CrossRef]
8. Hirano, M.; Yoshida, T.; Tanaka, S.; Hibi, S. Sulcus vocalis: Functional aspects. *Ann. Otol. Rhinol. Laryngol.* **1990**, *99 Pt 1*, 679–683. [CrossRef]
9. Dailey, S.H.; Spanou, K.; Zeitels, S.M. The evaluation of benign glottic lesions: Rigid telescopic stroboscopy versus suspension microlaryngoscopy. *J. Voice* **2007**, *21*, 112–118. [CrossRef]
10. Akbulut, S.; Altintas, H.; Oguz, H. Videolaryngostroboscopy versus microlaryngoscopy for the diagnosis of benign vocal cord lesions: A prospective clinical study. *Eur. Arch. Otorhinolaryngol.* **2015**, *272*, 131–136. [CrossRef]
11. Yildiz, M.G.; Sagiroglu, S.; Bilal, N.; Kara, I.; Orhan, I.; Doganer, A. Assessment of Subjective and Objective Voice Analysis According to Types of Sulcus Vocalis. *J. Voice* **2021**, in press. [CrossRef]
12. Dailey, S.H.; Ford, C.N. Surgical management of sulcus vocalis and vocal fold scarring. *Otolaryngol. Clin. N. Am.* **2006**, *39*, 23–42. [CrossRef]
13. Rajasudhakar, R. Effect of voice therapy in sulcus vocalis: A single case study. *S. Afr. J. Commun. Disord.* **2016**, *63*, e1–e5. [CrossRef]
14. Miaśkiewicz, B.; Szkiełkowska, A.; Gos, E.; Panasiewicz, A.; Włodarczyk, E.; Skarżyński, P.H. Pathological sulcus vocalis: Treatment approaches and voice outcomes in 36 patients. *Eur. Arch. Otorhinolaryngol.* **2018**, *275*, 2763–2771. [CrossRef]
15. Su, C.Y.; Tsai, S.S.; Chiu, J.F.; Cheng, C.A. Medialization laryngoplasty with strap muscle transposition for vocal fold atrophy with or without sulcus vocalis. *Laryngoscope* **2004**, *114*, 1106–1112. [CrossRef]
16. Saraniti, C.; Chianetta, E.; Greco, G.; Mat Lazim, N.; Verro, B. The Impact of Narrow-band Imaging on the Pre- and Intra-operative Assessments of Neoplastic and Preoplastic Laryngeal Lesions. A Systematic Review. *Int. Arch. Otorhinolaryngol.* **2021**, *25*, e471–e478. [CrossRef]
17. Hwang, C.S.; Lee, H.J.; Ha, J.G.; Cho, C.I.; Kim, N.H.; Hong, H.J.; Choi, H.S. Use of pulsed dye laser in the treatment of sulcus vocalis. *Otolaryngol. Head Neck Surg.* **2013**, *148*, 804–809. [CrossRef]
18. Verro, B.; Greco, G.; Chianetta, E.; Saraniti, C. Management of Early Glottic Cancer Treated by CO_2 Laser According to Surgical-Margin Status: A Systematic Review of the Literature. *Int. Arch. Otorhinolaryngol.* **2021**, *25*, e301–e308. [CrossRef]
19. Sung, C.K.; Tsao, G.J. Single-operator flexible nasolaryngoscopy-guided transthyrohyoid vocal fold injections. *Ann. Otol. Rhinol. Laryngol.* **2013**, *122*, 9–14. [CrossRef]
20. Kishimoto, Y.; Welham, N.V.; Hirano, S. Implantation of atelocollagen sheet for vocal fold scar. *Curr. Opin. Otolaryngol. Head Neck Surg.* **2010**, *18*, 507–511. [CrossRef]
21. Ford, C.N.; Bless, D.M. Selected problems treated by vocal fold injection of collagen. *Am. J. Otolaryngol* **1993**, *14*, 257–261. [CrossRef] [PubMed]
22. Neuenschwander, M.C.; Sataloff, R.T.; Abaza, M.M.; Hawkshaw, M.J.; Reiter, D.; Spiegel, J.R. Management of vocal fold scar with autologous fat implantation: Perceptual results. *J. Voice* **2001**, *15*, 295–304. [CrossRef] [PubMed]
23. Sataloff, R.T.; Spiegel, J.R.; Hawkshaw, M.; Rosen, D.C.; Heuer, R.J. Autologous fat implantation for vocal fold scar: A preliminary report. *J. Voice* **1997**, *11*, 238–246. [CrossRef] [PubMed]
24. Tsunoda, K.; Kondou, K.; Kaga, K.; Niimi, S.; Baer, T.; Nishiyama, K.; Hirose, H. Autologous transplantation of fascia into the vocal fold: Long-term result of type-1 transplantation and the future. *Laryngoscope* **2005**, *115 Pt 2*, 1–10. [CrossRef] [PubMed]
25. Eckley, C.A.; Corvo, M.A.; Yoshimi, R.; Swensson, J.; Duprat Ade, C. Unsuspected intraoperative finding of structural abnormalities associated with vocal fold polyps. *J. Voice* **2010**, *24*, 623–625. [CrossRef] [PubMed]
26. Saraniti, C.; Gallina, S.; Verro, B. NBI and Laryngeal Papillomatosis: A Diagnostic Challenge: A Systematic Review. *Int. J. Environ. Res. Public Health* **2022**, *19*, 8716. [CrossRef]
27. Sünter, A.V.; Kırgezen, T.; Yiğit, Ö.; Çakır, M. The association of sulcus vocalis and benign vocal cord lesions: Intraoperative findings. *Eur. Arch. Otorhinolaryngol.* **2019**, *276*, 3165–3171. [CrossRef]
28. Eckley, C.A.; Swensson, J.; Duprat Ade, C.; Donati, F.; Costa, H.O. Incidence of structural vocal fold abnormalities associated with vocal fold polyps. *Rev. Bras. Otorrinolaringol.* **2008**, *74*, 508–511. [CrossRef]
29. Carmel-Neiderman, N.N.; Wasserzug, O.; Ziv-Baran, T.; Oestreicher-Kedem, Y. Coexisting Vocal Fold Polyps and Sulcus Vocalis: Coincidence or Coexistence? Characteristics of 14 Patients. *J. Voice* **2018**, *32*, 239–243. [CrossRef]

30. Byeon, H.K.; Kim, J.H.; Kwon, J.H.; Jo, K.H.; Hong, H.J.; Choi, H.S. Clinical characteristics of vocal polyps with underlying sulcus vocalis. *J. Voice* **2013**, *27*, 632–635. [CrossRef]
31. Martins, R.H.; Silva, R.; Ferreira, D.M.; Dias, N.H. Sulcus vocalis: Probable genetic etiology. Report of four cases in close relatives. *Braz. J. Otorhinolaryngol.* **2007**, *73*, 573. [CrossRef]
32. Martins, R.H.; Gonçalves, T.M.; Neves, D.S.; Fracalossi, T.A.; Tavares, E.L.; Moretti-Ferreira, D. Sulcus vocalis: Evidence for autosomal dominant inheritance. *Genet. Mol. Res.* **2011**, *10*, 3163–3168. [CrossRef]
33. Nakayama, M.; Ford, C.N.; Brandenburg, J.H.; Bless, D.M. Sulcus vocalis in laryngeal cancer: A histopathologic study. *Laryngoscope* **1994**, *104 Pt 1*, 16–24. [CrossRef]
34. Shih, J.H.; Fay, M.P. Pearson's chi-square test and rank correlation inferences for clustered data. *Biometrics* **2017**, *73*, 822–834. [CrossRef]
35. Friedrich, G.; Dikkers, F.G.; Arens, C.; Remacle, M.; Hess, M.; Giovanni, A.; Duflo, S.; Hantzakos, A.; Bachy, V.; Gugatschka, M. Vocal fold scars: Current concepts and future directions. Consensus report of the Phonosurgery Committee of the European Laryngological Society. *Eur. Arch. Otorhinolaryngol.* **2013**, *270*, 2491–2507. [CrossRef]
36. Pontes, P.; Behlau, M.; Gonçalves, I. Alterações estruturais mínimas da laringe (AEM): Considerações básicas. *Acta AWHO* **1994**, *13*, 2–6.
37. Zhou, C.; Zhang, L.; Wu, Y.; Zhang, X.; Wu, D.; Tao, Z. Effects of Sulcus Vocalis Depth on Phonation in Three-Dimensional Fluid-Structure Interaction Laryngeal Models. *Appl. Bionics Biomech.* **2021**, *2021*, 6662625. [CrossRef]
38. Varelas, E.A.; Paddle, P.M.; Franco, R.A., Jr.; Husain, I.A. Identifying Type III Sulcus: Patient Characteristics and Endoscopic Findings. *Otolaryngol. Head Neck Surg.* **2020**, *163*, 1240–1243. [CrossRef]
39. Sato, K.; Hirano, M. Electron microscopic investigation of sulcus vocalis. *Ann. Otol. Rhinol. Laryngol.* **1998**, *107*, 56–60. [CrossRef]
40. Soares, A.B.; Moares, B.T.; Araújo, A.N.B.; de Biase, N.G.; Lucena, J.A. Laryngeal and Vocal Characterization of Asymptomatic Adults with Sulcus Vocalis. *Int. Arch. Otorhinolaryngol.* **2019**, *23*, e331–e337. [CrossRef]
41. Tsou, Y.A.; Tien, V.H.C.; Chen, S.H.; Shih, L.C.; Lin, T.C.; Chiu, C.J.; Chang, W.D. Autologous Fat Plus Platelet-Rich Plasma versus Autologous Fat Alone on Sulcus Vocalis. *J. Clin. Med.* **2022**, *11*, 725. [CrossRef]
42. Tan, S.H.; Sombuntham, P. Narrow band imaging for sulcus vocalis-an often missed diagnosis. *QJM* **2023**, *116*, 69–70. [CrossRef]
43. Desuter, G.; de Cock de Rameyen, D.; Boucquey, D. The "lake road sign": Another way to track the sulcus vocalis. *Ear Nose Throat J.* **2016**, *95*, 473. [CrossRef]
44. Lim, J.Y.; Kim, J.; Choi, S.H.; Kim, K.M.; Kim, Y.H.; Kim, H.S.; Choi, H.S. Sulcus configurations of vocal folds during phonation. *Acta Oto-Laryngol.* **2009**, *129*, 1127–1135. [CrossRef]

Disclaimer/Publisher's Note: The statements, opinions and data contained in all publications are solely those of the individual author(s) and contributor(s) and not of MDPI and/or the editor(s). MDPI and/or the editor(s) disclaim responsibility for any injury to people or property resulting from any ideas, methods, instructions or products referred to in the content.

Article

Benign Paroxysmal Positional Vertigo Is Associated with an Increased Risk for Migraine Diagnosis: A Nationwide Population-Based Cohort Study

I-An Shih [1,2,3], Chung-Y. Hsu [4], Tsai-Chung Li [1,5,*] and Shuu-Jiun Wang [6,7,8,9,*]

1. Department of Public Health, College of Public Health, China Medical University, Taichung 404327, Taiwan
2. Department of Neurology, Ching Chyuan Hospital, Taichung 428433, Taiwan
3. Premium Healthcare Center, Chung Shan Medical University Hospital, Taichung 402306, Taiwan
4. Graduate Institute of Biomedical Sciences, China Medical University, Taichung 406040, Taiwan
5. Department of Healthcare Administration, College of Medical and Health Science, Asia University, Taichung 413305, Taiwan
6. Department of Neurology, Neurological Institute, Taipei Veterans General Hospital, Taipei 11217, Taiwan
7. Department of Neurology, National Yang-Ming Chiao Tung University School of Medicine, Taipei 11217, Taiwan
8. Institute of Brain Science, National Yang-Ming Chiao Tung University School of Medicine, Taipei 11217, Taiwan
9. Brain Research Center, National Yang-Ming Chiao Tung University School of Medicine, Taipei 11217, Taiwan
* Correspondence: tcli@mail.cmu.edu.tw (T.-C.L.); sjwang@vghtpe.gov.tw (S.-J.W.)

Abstract: Previous studies reported an increased risk of benign paroxysmal positional vertigo (BPPV) in patients with migraine. Hence, we aimed to assess the risk of migraine in patients with BPPV. This cohort study was conducted using the Taiwan National Health Insurance Research Database. The BPPV cohort consisted of patients aged <45 years with a diagnosis of BPPV between 2000 and 2009. An age- and sex-matched comparison group free from a history of BPPV or migraine was selected. All cases were followed up from 1 January 2000 to 31 December 2010 or until death or a diagnosis of migraine. The baseline demographic characteristics in both groups were compared using Student's t-test and the chi-square test. Cox proportional hazards regression analysis was used to estimate the hazard ratio for migraine in the BPPV cohort compared with the comparison group after adjustment for age, sex, and comorbidities. Notably, 117 of the 1386 participants with BPPV and 146 of the 5544 participants without BPPV developed migraine. After adjustment for age, sex, and comorbidities, BPPV showed an adjusted hazard ratio indicating a 2.96-fold increased risk of migraine (95% confidence interval: 2.30–3.80, $p < 0.001$). We found that BPPV is associated with an increased risk of a migraine diagnosis.

Keywords: benign paroxysmal positional vertigo; migraine; cohort study

1. Introduction

Benign paroxysmal positional vertigo (BPPV) is the most common cause of vertigo. A study reported that the lifetime prevalence rate of BPPV is 2.4% [1]. Idiopathic BPPV is more prevalent in older adults than in younger adults, with a peak onset between 50 and 60 years. It is also more prevalent in females than males, with a male-to-female ratio of 1:2–1:3. The typical symptom of BPPV is recurrent episodes of vertigo lasting for ≤1 min provoked by head movement. While each episode is brief, vertigo typically recurs in weeks without therapy [2] and is thought to be caused by the displacement of otoliths from otolithic organs into the semicircular canals [3,4]. However, the cause of the otolith displacement remains unknown. The Dix–Hallpike maneuver and head-roll test induce nystagmus in patients with suspected BPPV. After a clinical diagnosis of BPPV, Epley's canalith-repositioning maneuver is used to treat patients immediately.

Migraine is the second most prevalent neurologic disorder, with a male-to-female ratio of 1:3 [5]. The 1-year prevalence rate of migraine was reported to be 9.1% in Taiwan [6]. The prevalence of migraine in males is highest in the age range of 25–29 years (8.3%), whereas it is highest in females in the age range of 30–34 years (21.1%). Most migraine diagnoses are made clinically according to the International Classification of Headache Disorders, 2nd Edition, 2004 [7]. With core symptoms and adequate follow-up time, a clinical diagnosis of migraine is primarily made in an outpatient setting. However, physicians should consider secondary headache disorder if the onset of migraine is noted after the age of 50 years [5,7]. Migraine is now a manageable disease entity with much evidence supporting preventive and abortive treatments [8]. Among the various subtypes of migraine, vestibular migraine introduced in the International Classification of Headache Disorders appendix, 3rd Edition, stands out with its presentation of vestibular symptoms lasting between 5 min and 72 h [9]. The duration of vestibular migraine symptoms is longer than that of BPPV [10,11]. Characteristic features of migrainous positional vertigo include short duration, frequent recurrence, onset in early life, migrainous symptoms during episodes of positional vertigo, and atypical positional nystagmus [11–15]. However, the vestibular migraine criteria are for research purposes, and better scientific evidence is warranted before vestibular migraine can be formally accepted.

As per Kayan et al., patients with migraine presented with vertigo three times more often than patients with tension-type headaches (26.5% vs. 7.8%) [16]. Dizziness and vertigo occur in 20–30% and 25–26% of patients with a primary complaint of migraine, respectively [17]. Hence, some clinical questions, such as "Do patients suffer BPPV before migraine onset?" and "If a patient had been diagnosed with BPPV, will the exposure to BPPV increase the risk of migraine in the patient?" arose. Even with multiple cross-sectional studies showing the association between migraine and BPPV, the main conundrum is that both disease entities are very frequent in the general population. However, there seems to be no cohort study investigating the incidence of migraine in adults with BPPV. Among the various types of vertigo and relatively nonspecific dizziness, we chose BPPV as the exposure in this cohort study because BPPV is the most common type of vertigo. This study aimed to investigate the risk of migraine in patients with BPPV using a retrospective cohort study design and a population-based research database.

2. Materials and Methods

2.1. National Health Insurance Research Database

The National Health Insurance Research Database (NHIRD) is a comprehensive database covering approximately 100% of the population in Taiwan. All information that would expose a person's identity had been de-identified. The regulations from the Bureau of National Health Insurance (NHI) and the National Health Research Institute maintain the confidentiality of data. The 2000 Longitudinal Health Insurance Database (LHID) is a data subset randomly sampling 1 million people from the population between 1996 and 2010. The LHID used the International Classification of Disease, Ninth Revision, Clinical Modification (ICD-9-CM) to record disease entities. It is openly provided to researchers in Taiwan for scientific and epidemiological purposes. It includes the medical claims data for outpatient and inpatient services. The full ethical privacy of this study was approved by the Research Ethics Committee of China Medical University, and it was exempt from full review. This study used the outpatient records in the NHIRD as the data source.

2.2. Study Population

Given the background knowledge of the peak age of migraine onset being 25–35 years of age in Taiwan and the high possibility of misclassification bias in migraine diagnosis in patients >50 years, we collected data on newly diagnosed BPPV (ICD-9-CM code 386.11) cases between 2000 and 2009 from the LHID, with the baseline age being <45 years. First, patients with a previous diagnosis of migraine were excluded to avoid reverse causality.

Then, we defined the index date of the BPPV case as the date of the initial BPPV diagnosis. Next, the date, month, and year of the index date of the selected case were assigned to the comparison cohort. Afterward, we adopted an individual matching method using age and sex at a ratio of 4:1 to randomly select individuals without a history of BPPV or migraine before the index date.

2.3. Baseline Characteristics

We included comorbidities before the index date as the baseline comorbidities, including hypertension (ICD-9-CM codes 401–405), diabetes mellitus (ICD-9-CM code 250), hyperlipidemia (ICD-9-CM code 272), anxiety (ICD-9-CM codes 300.0, 300.2, 300.3, 308.3, and 309.81), and depression (ICD-9-CM codes 296.2–296.3, 300.4 and 311), to further adjust for possible confounding factors. The comorbidities were selected because hypertension, diabetes mellitus, and hyperlipidemia are known risk factors for BPPV and BPPV recurrence [18,19], and anxiety and depression are known comorbidities in migraine [20].

2.4. Outcome

The primary outcome was the occurrence of migraine, defined as the first ambulatory visit associated with an ICD-9-CM code of 346, during the follow-up period. Both cohorts were followed up until 31 December 2010, or until death or the diagnosis of migraine.

2.5. Statistical Analysis

For descriptive statistical analysis, we used the chi-squared test and Student's t-test to compare baseline demographic characteristics between the BPPV and matched control groups. We calculated the cumulative incidence of migraine for each group by dividing the total number of migraine events by the total sum of the follow-up person-years (per 10,000 person-years). We used the Cox proportional hazards regression model to analyze the overall, age-specific, sex-specific, and each comorbidity-specific risks of developing migraine associated with BPPV. Furthermore, we calculated the adjusted hazard ratio (aHR) of migraine presenting with a 95% confidence interval (CI) for the BPPV group after adjusting for age, sex, and comorbidities.

The statistical program SAS 9.3 (SAS Institute Inc., Cary, NC, USA) was used for all statistical analyses. The Kaplan-Meier estimate for measuring the cumulative incidence in both groups was calculated using R software (R Foundation for Statistical Computing, Vienna, Austria). Then, we compared the differences in the cumulative incidence curves between the two groups using the log-rank test. Statistical significance was set at $p < 0.05$ in a two-tailed test.

3. Results

3.1. Baseline Demographic Characteristics in the Study Groups

Within the 11-year study period, 1386 patients without previous a BPPV or migraine history who had a baseline age <45 years were diagnosed with BPPV. Based on individual matching using age and sex at a 4:1 ratio, 5544 patients were included in the control group after excluding those with a history of migraine or BPPV before the index date. The distribution of age and sex was similar between the two groups. In both cohorts, the mean age was 33.2 years. In addition, both cohorts had a female predominance (68.0%).

The baseline demographic status and comorbidities between the BPPV and control groups are shown in Table 1. The mean follow-up duration was 6.23 and 6.46 years in the BPPV and control groups, respectively. The prevalence rate of all comorbidities, including hypertension, diabetes mellitus, hyperlipidemia, anxiety, and depression, was considerably higher in the BPPV group than in the control group.

Table 1. Baseline demographic status of patients within the BPPV and control groups.

Characteristics		BPPV Group n = 1386	Control Group n = 5544	p-Value
		No. (%)	No. (%)	
Mean age, years (SD) *		33.2 (8.84)	33.1 (8.89)	0.74
Sex				>0.99
	Female	942 (68.0)	3768 (68.0)	
	Male	444 (32.0)	1776 (32.0)	
Comorbidity				
	Hypertension	134 (9.67)	221 (3.99)	<0.0001
	DM	44 (3.17)	83 (1.59)	<0.0001
	Hyperlipidemia	124 (8.95)	257 (4.64)	<0.0001
	Anxiety	234 (16.9)	292 (5.27)	<0.0001
	Depression	105 (7.58)	166 (2.99)	<0.0001

* Results are according to Student's *t*-test. Abbreviations: BPPV: benign paroxysmal positional vertigo; DM: diabetes mellitus.

3.2. Comparison of the Incidence of Migraine Diagnosis between the BPPV and Control Groups

Table 2 shows the comparison of migraine incidence between BPPV and matched control patients. Within the 11-year follow-up period, 117 (1.35%) and 146 (0.41%) patients had migraine in the BPPV and control groups, respectively. The overall cumulative incidence of migraine was 3.31-fold higher in the BPPV group than in the matched control group (135.4 vs. 40.8 per 10,000 person-years). After adjusting for demographic characteristics, the BPPV cohort had a 2.96-fold higher risk of migraine than the matched control cohort (aHR: 2.96, 95% CI: 2.30–3.80).

Table 2. Incidence of migraine in the BPPV and comparison groups using multivariate Cox proportional hazards regression analysis.

Characteristics	Patient with BPPV; n = 1386		Matched Cohort; n = 5544		Adjusted HR (95% CI)	p-Value
	Migraine, No.	Per 10,000 Person-Years	Migraine, No.	Per 10,000 Person-Years		
Total	117	135.4	146	40.8	2.96 (2.30–3.80)	<0.001

Model adjusted for age, sex, hypertension, diabetes mellitus, hyperlipidemia, anxiety, and depression. Abbreviations: BPPV: benign paroxysmal positional vertigo; HR: hazard ratio; CI: confidence interval.

As shown in Figure 1, the BPPV group had a higher cumulative incidence of migraine than the matched control group, with the log-rank test showing the difference ($p < 0.001$).

3.3. Risk Factors for Migraine in Patients with BPPV

Using Cox proportional hazards regression analysis, a markedly higher hazard ratio of having a migraine in this specific BPPV sample and matched control cohorts was observed in females (aHR: 2.91; 95% CI: 2.30–3.80), those with hyperlipidemia (aHR:1.77; 95% CI: 1.16–2.70), and those with anxiety (aHR: 1.49; 95% CI: 1.03–2.14) (Table 3).

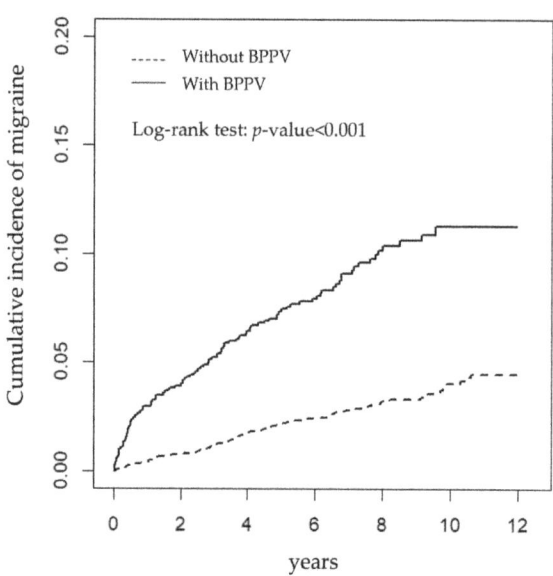

Figure 1. The cumulative incidence of newly diagnosed migraine using Kaplan-Meier survival analysis in patients with (solid line) and without (dashed line) benign paroxysmal positional vertigo (BPPV).

Table 3. Incidence of migraine and multivariate Cox proportional hazards regression analysis measures of hazard ratio for the study cohort.

Variable	Event	PYs	Rate	Crude HR (95% CI)	Adjusted HR (95% CI)
Age group					
<20	15	4252	35.3	Ref	Ref
20–34	110	17,069	64.4	1.82 (1.06–3.12)	1.60 (0.93–2.76)
35–45	138	23,148	59.6	1.70 (0.99–2.89)	1.34 (0.78–2.31)
Sex					
Female	226	30,263	74.7	2.86 (2.02–4.05)	2.91 (2.05–4.13)
Male	37	14,207	26.0	Ref	Ref
Hypertension					
No	237	42,242	56.1	Ref	Ref
Yes	26	2228	116.7	2.09 (1.39–3.13)	1.50 (0.97–2.32)
DM					
No	259	43,611	59.4	Ref	Ref
Yes	4	858	46.6	0.79 (0.29–2.11)	0.47 (0.17–1.29)
Hyperlipidemia					
No	236	42,088	56.1	Ref	Ref
Yes	27	2381	113.4	2.01 (1.35–2.99)	1.77 (1.16–2.70)
Anxiety					
No	221	41,442	53.3	Ref	Ref
Yes	42	3028	138.7	2.54 (1.83–3.54)	1.49 (1.03–2.14)
Depression					
No	243	42,940	56.6	Ref	Ref
Yes	20	1529	130.8	2.25 (1.43–3.56)	1.30 (0.80–2.12)

Model adjusted for age, sex, hypertension, DM, hyperlipidemia, anxiety, and depression. Rate is the incidence rate per 10,000 person-years. Abbreviations: CI: confidence intervals; DM: diabetes mellitus; HR: hazard ratio; PYs: person-years.

3.4. Subgroup Analysis of Migraine Risk

The subgroup analysis showed that an increased migraine risk was associated with age, sex, hypertension, diabetes mellitus, hyperlipidemia, anxiety, and depression (Table 4). However, sex may be associated with migraine occurrence in patients with BPPV. Male BPPV patients may have a more increased hazard ratio for developing migraine than female patients with BPPV. The migraine incidence in control males was 10.5 per 10,000 person-years, approximately one-fourth of the mean incidence (40.8 per 10,000 person-years) in the whole control group. This may amplify the increased aHR in the subgroup analysis of males compared with females.

Table 4. Subgroup analysis of migraine in the BPPV and age- and sex-matched control cohorts.

Comorbidity	Comparison Group			BPPV Group			Adjusted HR (95% CI)	p for Interaction
	Event	PYs	Rate	Event	PYs	Rate		
Age group								0.68
<20	9	3431	26.2	6	820	73.1	2.65 (0.92–7.66)	
20–34	62	13,749	45.1	48	3319	144.6	3.00 (2.03–4.44)	
≥35	75	18,645	40.2	63	4502	139.9	2.96 (2.09–4.20)	
Sex								0.003
Female	134	24,394	54.9	92	5868	156.8	2.50 (1.90–3.29)	
Male	12	11,432	10.5	25	2774	90.1	8.10 (3.99–16.4)	
Hypertension								0.96
No	137	34,412	39.8	100	7830	127.7	2.92 (2.24–3.81)	
Yes	9	1415	63.6	17	813	209.2	2.75 (1.18–6.42)	
DM								0.15
No	143	35,260	40.6	116	8352	138.9	3.01 (2.34–3.88)	
Yes	3	567	52.9	1	291	34.4	0.99 (0.10–9.79)	
Hyperlipidemia								0.06
No	131	34,244	38.3	105	7844	133.9	3.17 (2.43–4.13)	
Yes	15	1583	94.8	12	799	150.3	1.60 (0.74–3.45)	
Anxiety								0.71
No	135	34,170	39.5	86	7272	118.3	2.85 (2.16–3.75)	
Yes	11	1656	66.4	31	1371	226.1	3.67 (1.83–7.35)	
Depression								0.84
No	140	34,912	40.1	103	8028	128.3	2.88 (2.22–3.75)	
Yes	6	914	65.6	14	615	227.6	3.50 (1.31–9.39)	

Model adjusted for age, sex, hypertension, DM, hyperlipidemia, anxiety, and depression. Rate is the incidence rate per 10,000 person-years. Abbreviations: BPPV: benign paroxysmal positional vertigo; CI: confidence interval; DM: diabetes mellitus; HR: hazard ratio; PYs: person-years.

3.5. Sensitivity Test

Further analysis of migraine risk stratified by different specialties diagnosing BPPV is presented in Table 5; this demonstrated a consistently higher migraine risk in the BPPV group stratified by different specialties making the BPPV diagnosis.

Table 5. Migraine risk stratified by different specialties diagnosing BPPV.

Variable	N	Event	PYs	Rate	Crude HR (95% CI)	Adjusted HR (95% CI)
Comparison cohort	5544	146	35,827	40.8	Ref	Ref
BPPV cohort						
Neurology	149	8	882	90.7	2.19 (1.08–4.47)	2.05 (1.00–4.19)
Otolaryngology	383	24	2175	110.3	2.65 (1.72–4.08)	2.49 (1.61–3.85)
Family medicine	214	18	1270	141.8	3.42 (2.09–5.58)	2.85 (1.73–4.69)
Internal medicine	310	33	2169	152.2	3.81 (2.61–5.57)	3.39 (2.30–5.00)
Others	203	18	1229	146.5	3.56 (2.18–5.81)	3.12 (1.90–5.12)

Model adjusted for age, sex, hypertension, diabetes mellitus, hyperlipidemia, anxiety, and depression. Rate: incidence rate per 10,000 person-years. Abbreviations: BPPV: benign paroxysmal positional vertigo; CI: confidence interval; HR: hazard ratio; PYs: person-years.

4. Discussion

This study mainly demonstrated that the risk of migraine was 2.96 times higher in the BPPV cohort than in the age- and sex-matched control cohort after adjusting for age, sex, and comorbidities. The incidence of migraine diagnosis was 135.4 per 10,000 person-years in patients with BPPV, whereas it was 40.8 in the age- and sex-matched control group. Furthermore, a higher risk of migraine was associated with three factors in patients aged <45 years and with a BPPV history: female sex (aHR: 2.91), hyperlipidemia (aHR: 1.77), and anxiety (aHR: 1.49). To our knowledge, this study is the first population-based cohort study to show that BPPV is associated with an increased risk of migraine.

Our study has various clinical implications. The atypical earlier onset age of BPPV among patients in clinical settings should prompt physicians to note migraine-related history, especially in female patients, those with a history of hyperlipidemia, or those with a history of anxiety. This is because these factors were independently associated with a higher migraine risk in patients with BPPV.

We limited the inclusion baseline age of patients to <45 years for three reasons. First, it avoids misclassification bias in the diagnosis of migraine in patients >50 years [10]. Second, the age specification limits the effect of baseline comorbidities and other unmeasured confounding factors leading to unmeasured selection bias and confounding regarding the risk of migraine between the two groups. Third, based on the 11-year timeframe of the database research and the peak age of migraine prevalence in males and females being 25–29 and 30–34 years, respectively, in Taiwan [6], it is reasonable to establish an age specification of <45 years to evaluate the age range associated with the highest risk as that between 25 and 34 years for the diagnosis of migraine in the included BPPV and age- and sex-matched control groups.

The mean baseline age of the BPPV and matched control cohorts were 33.2 and 33.1 years, respectively. However, this is not the typical prevalence age of patients with BPPV. Therefore, the number of patients in our BPPV group was relatively low. However, the mean baseline age is in the age range (25–34 years) of migraine peak prevalence in Taiwan. Furthermore, the male: female ratio was approximately 1:2, which is relatively consistent with the general epidemiological sex ratio of patients with BPPV. Comorbidities such as hypertension, diabetes mellitus, hyperlipidemia, anxiety, and depression were notably more common in the BPPV group than in the control group. While other methods, such as propensity score matching, may adjust the possible baseline demographic differences at the beginning of sample selection to reduce the selection bias and impact of confounding factors, the representative control group will also be changed from an age- and sex-matched general population sample to a more comorbidity-bound population sample. In this study, we aimed to compare the risk of migraine between patients with BPPV and a more general population to increase the external validity of the result.

Because our study showed a lower prevalence rate of migraine than the epidemiological study, we changed our paper title from "migraine" to "migraine diagnosis." A previous study in Taiwan showed a 1-year migraine prevalence rate of 9.1% [6]. In our study, the incidence of migraine was 135.4 per 10,000 person-years in the BPPV group, whereas it was 40.8 in the age- and sex-matched control cohort. The 1-year prevalence rate of migraine in both cohorts was 1.35% and 0.41%, respectively, during the study period. This is far below the expected prevalence rate of migraine.

There are several epidemiological reports associating migraine with BPPV. However, to the best of our knowledge, there are neither cohort nor case-control studies investigating migraine risk in patients with BPPV. Nevertheless, a few cross-sectional studies have reported on the associations between migraine and BPPV. In a cross-sectional study by Lee et al., migraine is associated with BPPV with an odds ratio of 2.05 compared with the control group ($p < 0.001$) [21]. Another cross-sectional study showed that patients with BPPV had a three times higher historical rate of migraine than the general population and a higher family history of migraine (58.4% vs. 12.6%) and episodic vertigo (44.9% vs. 18%) in patients with BPPV than in patients with other dizziness and vertigo [22]. However, a cross-sectional study showed no significant association between migraine and BPPV in 508 patients in balance clinics [23]. Two population-based cohort studies investigated BPPV occurrence in patients with migraine. The first study, in Taiwan, showed a 2.03-fold higher risk of having BPPV in patients with migraine than in the age-, sex-, and comorbidities-matched controls (incidence rate ratio: 2.03; 95% CI: 1.41–2.97; $p < 0.001$) [24]. In the study with the same database as ours, no age specification was given due to the natural course of migraine peak age (25–34 years), followed by BPPV peak age (50–60 years). The second study, which had a larger sample size and a longer follow-up duration and was conducted in Korea, showed a 2.54-fold higher incidence of BPPV in migraine patients (aHR, 2.54; 95% CI: 2.41–2.68) [25]. The longer duration may more likely expose the patients in the migraine group between 50–60 years to BPPV. This may increase the likelihood of BPPV occurrence in the Korean study. Table 6 provides a general overview of the findings on the associations between BPPV and migraine in previous cohort studies.

Table 6. Associations between BPPV and migraine in cohort studies.

Author Year Location Reference	Exposure Outcome	Matching Method	Matching Factors	Disease Coding	No. of Cases	Confounding Factors Adjusted	Brief Finding on Association
Chu 2015 Taiwan [24]	Migraine BPPV	1:1 PSM	PSM by age, sex, DM, HTN, heart failure, COPD, asthma, CKD, CAD, CVD, hyperlipidemia, cirrhosis, and autoimmune disease	ICD-9	8266 with migraine 8266 PSM controls	PSM	IRR of BPPV: 2.03 in migraine (95% CI: 1.41–2.97)
Kim 2019 Korea [25]	Migraine BPPV	1:4 individual matching	Age group, sex, income group, region of residence, and medical history of HTN, DM, and dyslipidemia	ICD-10	40,682 migraine, 162,728 controls	Matching factors and history of ischemic heart disease cerebral stroke, and depression	Migraine increased risk of BPPV (aHR: 2.54; 95% CI, 2.41–2.68)
Shih 2023 Taiwan (this study)	BPPV Migraine	1:4 individual matching	Age and sex	ICD-9	1386 with BPPV 5544 controls	Age, sex, HTN, DM, hyperlipidemia, anxiety, and depression	BPPV increased risk of migraine (aHR: 2.96, 95% CI: 2.30–3.80)

Abbreviations: aHR: adjusted hazard ratio; BPPV: benign paroxysmal positional vertigo; CI: confidence interval; CAD: coronary artery disease; CKD: chronic kidney disease; COPD: chronic obstructive pulmonary disease; CVD: cerebrovascular disease; DM: diabetes mellitus; HTN: hypertension; ICD-9: International Statistical Classification of Diseases and Related Health Problems 9th Revision; ICD-10: International Statistical Classification of Diseases and Related Health Problems 10th Revision; IRR: incidence rate ratio; PSM: propensity-score matching.

Many observational surveys, including case series, have reported the association between BPPV and migraine [26–31]. The association between BPPV and migraine is not always consistent due to different study populations. Generally, these studies presented what is observed in the vertigo clinic, that patients with BPPV have a higher migraine prevalence. Patients with BPPV and a history of migraine tended to be younger with a female predominance. As presented by Faralli et al., the mean age was younger in patients with BPPV and migraine, and the recurrence rate of >4 documented episodes of BPPV was higher than in patients with BPPV without headache or migraine (39 vs. 53 years and 19.4% vs. 7.3%). No significant difference was observed in the number of maneuvers needed to achieve recovery between the two groups [27]. In headache clinics, neurologists seldom find patients with migraine with a history of BPPV [16,32]. Instead, in interviewing the patients, complaints of dizziness and vertigo existed. Therefore, observational reports suggested a higher prevalence of vertigo in patients with classical migraine than in patients with common migraine, tension-type headaches, and cluster headaches (42%, 12%, 17%, and 14%, respectively) [32]. Another study reported a higher vertigo prevalence in migraine than in tension-type headache (26.5% vs. 7.8% $p < 0.001$) [16]. Interestingly, there was no difference in neurotologic abnormality in patients with migraine presenting with or without vestibular symptoms [33]. As noticed in the literature, neurologists found a higher prevalence of vertigo in patients with migraine than in patients with tension-type headaches. Moreover, otolaryngologists found a higher migraine history in patients with BPPV than other dizziness and vertigo. The lack of time sequence between migraine and BPPV in cross-sectional studies and the lack of control groups in case series studies are the main limitations of the study design. A cohort study is the better observational study design in this situation. Another summary of published cross-sectional studies and case series studies investigating associations between BPPV and migraine with the exclusion of vestibular migraine is presented in Table 7.

Table 7. Associations between BPPV and migraine in cross-sectional studies and case series studies.

Author Year Reference	Questionnaire Examination	Study Population	Major Finding
Uneri 2004 [22]	Motion sickness Migraine history FH of migraine FH of BPPV	477 BPPV 117 Control: other dizziness/vertigo	BPPV group vs. control group: FH of migraine: 58.4% vs. 12.6% FH of episodic vertigo: 44.9% vs. 18%
Pollak 2014 [26]	History of headache History of BPPV Background disease	53 headache with BPPV 52 age/sex-matched BPPV without headache	No difference in history of headache, history of BPPV, or background disease
Faralli 2014 [27]	Mean age Recurrence rate of BPPV	77 BPPV with migraine 109 BPPV without migraine or with other kinds of headache	Mean age in patients with BPPV and migraine compared with other kinds of headache (39 vs. 53 years) High recurrence rate of BPPV (>4) documented episodes (19.4% vs. 7.3%).
Yetiser 2015 [28]	Migraine	263 BPPV patients	32 patients had migraine (11.4%). Higher female: male ratio in BPPV with migraine vs. BPPV without migraine (4.2:1 vs. 1.3:1). No difference in mean age
Teixido 2017 [23]	Migraine	508 Balance clinic	No significant association between migraine and BPPV
Hilton 2020 [29]	Migraine	1481 BPPV patients	The prevalence of migraine among the study sample was 25.8%. Female gender, prior history of BPPV, younger age, and lack of diabetes were independently associated with the concurrent comorbidity of BPPV and migraine.
Lee 2021 [21]	BPPV and other vestibular symptoms	16,982 migraine 371,038 controls 103,699 non-migraine	Migraine: OR 2.05 for BPPV ($p < 0.001$). Non-migraine: OR 1.73 for BPPV ($p < 0.001$)
Grupta 2022 [30]	Migraine	100 BPV patients	34% with BPV with headache (including migraine), 10% with migraine
Kim 2022 [31]	Migraine	255 BPPV patients	44.7% had a history of migraine. Those with migraine had an earlier age of BPPV onset than individuals without migraine (60.2 vs. 65.4, $p = 0.0018$).

Abbreviations: BPPV: benign paroxysmal positional vertigo; BPV: benign positional vertigo; FH: family history; OR: odds ratio.

The pathophysiological association between migraine and BPPV remains unclear. Three mechanisms associating migraine with BPPV have been previously proposed. First, vasospasm caused by migraine may be responsible for vertigo or cochlear symptoms. Baloh postulated that ontological symptoms in patients with migraine might occur from vasospasm or a certain iron channel disorder [34]. Ishiyama et al. proposed that repeated vasospasm can influence the microvasculature of the inner ear [35]. Repeated vasospasm may stress and damage the vestibular cells, thus resulting in the dislodgement of otoconia from the macula. The suppression of inner-ear microvasculature further leads to cochlear symptoms, such as hearing loss and vestibular symptoms. This association mechanism was supported by a previous study that showed an increased incidence rate of sudden sensorineural hearing loss in patients with migraine [36]. Second, the effect of neuropeptides, such as substance P, neurokinin A, nitrous oxide, and calcitonin gene-related peptide (CGRP), may cause sudden sensorineural hearing loss in patients with BPPV. CGRP is a neuropeptide involved in the efferent synapses of hair cell organs, such as the cochlea, semicircular canal, and lateral line [37]. Deletion of CGRP in transgenic mice was associated with reduced suprathreshold cochlear nerve activity and decreased vestibulo–ocular reflex gain. The recent success of many CGRP-related medications for migraine implies that the vestibular system plays an essential role in the pathogenesis of migraine [8]. Third, the CAMERA study demonstrated that a combination of hypoperfusion and embolism is the most likely mechanism for posterior circulation infarction in migraine [38]. The relative hypoperfusion may result in vertigo, as noted in vertebra–basilar insufficiency [38,39]. A cross-sectional study demonstrated the possible association between vertebral artery abnormality and BPPV [40].

Benign paroxysmal vertigo of childhood is one of the periodic childhood syndromes commonly regarded as a precursor of migraine, as described in the International Classification of Headache Disorders, 3rd Edition [9]. In this study, the annual conversion rate from BPPV to migraine was low (1.35%), with an 11-year accumulation incidence of 8.4%. In benign paroxysmal vertigo of childhood, the accumulation incidence rate of migraine with an average follow-up duration of 18 years and 15.7 years was 33.3% and 21%, respectively [41,42]. Hence, we were not able to infer further whether BPPV is a precursor to migraine. Rather, we postulated that a shared pathophysiological relationship might exist. This study's result is also consistent with the previous notion that patients with acute migrainous vertigo develop central and peripheral vestibular dysfunctions [33].

This study has three major strengths. First, combined with the nationwide population-based cohort, the large sample size of one million citizens covered under the national health insurance in Taiwan and the 11-year adequate follow-up period for migraine occurrence provide enough power for differences between the two groups. Second, with the age specification of <45 years as the inclusion criterion, we tried to avoid a higher probability of migraine misclassification bias in the older population. Although some of the patients with migraine may present to the clinic after years of migraine suffering at age ≥ 50 years, we set the age specification not for definition purposes but rather for the need for validity. Moreover, with an age specification of <45 years in our study, the mean baseline age of both groups was 32 years. This was also good for migraine occurrence because migraine is a relatively early-onset disease entity with a peak onset age of 25–34 years in Taiwan. The 11-year follow-up period for migraine occurrence was adequate.

This study had some limitations. First, selection bias is prominent in our study, as shown in our baseline demographic state (Table 1), even with the baseline age specification of <45 years. Second, although known confounding factors, such as female sex, were controlled using a matching method, confounding is still a major source of bias in cohort studies because possible unknown confounders may exist. Third, misclassification of BPPV and migraine is still possible in this cohort study, even with the age specification to control the bias of inappropriate diagnosis of migraine in patients >50 years. However, it is worth noting that the differentiation of peripheral and central vertigo may occasionally be difficult in a clinical setting. In the case of BPPV, the difficulty may be ameliorated but not completely overcome. However, the lack of validation studies of BPPV in the database made this a serious limitation of our study. Finally, the severity, duration, and frequency of BPPV and migraine were not recorded in our database, and further exploration of their association was impossible.

5. Conclusions

Our study indicated a 2.96-fold higher risk of a migraine diagnosis in patients with BPPV than in age- and sex-matched controls in Taiwan. In addition, three other factors, including female sex, hyperlipidemia, and anxiety, were associated with an increased migraine diagnosis in this study.

Author Contributions: Conceptualization, I.-A.S., S.-J.W. and T.-C.L.; methodology, T.-C.L. and C.-Y.H.; software, C.-Y.H.; validation, I.-A.S. and S.-J.W.; formal analysis, I.-A.S.; investigation, I.-A.S.; resources, C.-Y.H.; data curation, C.-Y.H.; writing—original draft preparation, I.-A.S.; writing—review and editing, T.-C.L. and S.-J.W.; visualization, C.-Y.H.; supervision, S.-J.W. and T.-C.L.; project administration, S.-J.W. All authors have read and agreed to the published version of the manuscript.

Funding: This research received no external funding.

Institutional Review Board Statement: The study was conducted in accordance with the Declaration of Helsinki and approved by the Research Ethics Committee of China Medical University and Hospital (protocol code: CMUH104-REC2-115(CR-7), 27 May 2022).

Informed Consent Statement: Patient consent was waived as the data used in this study were deidentified and encrypted.

Data Availability Statement: The National Health Insurance Record Database is publicly available from the Taiwan National Health Institute. With academic or commercial requests, Taiwan citizens can have access to the research database.

Acknowledgments: We are grateful to the Health Data Science Center, China Medical University Hospital for providing administrative and technical support.

Conflicts of Interest: The authors declare no conflict of interest.

References

1. Kim, J.-S.; Zee, D.S. Clinical Practice. Benign paroxysmal positional vertigo. *N. Engl. J. Med.* **2014**, *370*, 1138–1147. [CrossRef] [PubMed]
2. von Brevern, M.; Bertholon, P.; Brandt, T.; Fife, T.; Imai, T.; Nuti, D.; Newman-Toker, D. Benign paroxysmal positional vertigo: Diagnostic criteria consensus document of the Committee for the Classification of Vestibular Disorders of the Bárány Society. *Acta Otorrinolaringol.* **2017**, *68*, 349–360. [CrossRef] [PubMed]
3. Welling, D.B.; Parnes, L.S.; O'Brien, B.; Bakaletz, L.O.; Brackmann, D.E.; Hinojosa, R. Particulate matter in the posterior semicircular canal. *Laryngoscope* **1997**, *107*, 90–94. [CrossRef] [PubMed]
4. Parnes, L.S.; McClure, J.A. Free-floating endolymph particles: A new operative finding during posterior semicircular canal occlusion. *Laryngoscope* **1992**, *102*, 988–992. [CrossRef] [PubMed]
5. Woldeamanuel, Y.W.; Cowan, R.P. Migraine affects 1 in 10 people worldwide featuring recent rise: A systematic review and meta-analysis of community-based studies involving 6 million participants. *J. Neurol. Sci.* **2017**, *372*, 307–315. [CrossRef]
6. Wang, S.J.; Fuh, J.L.; Young, Y.H.; Lu, S.R.; Shia, B.C. Prevalence of migraine in Taipei, Taiwan: A population-based survey. *Cephalalgia* **2000**, *20*, 566–572. [CrossRef]
7. Headache Classification Subcommittee of the International Headache Society The International Classification of Headache Disorders: 2nd Edition. *Cephalalgia* **2004**, *24* (Suppl. S1), 9–160. [CrossRef]
8. Ashina, M. Migraine. *N. Engl. J. Med.* **2020**, *383*, 1866–1876. [CrossRef]
9. Headache Classification Committee of the International Headache Society (IHS) the International Classification of Headache Disorders, 3rd Edition. *Cephalalgia* **2018**, *38*, 1–211. [CrossRef]
10. GBD 2016 Headache Collaborators Global, Regional, and National Burden of Migraine and Tension-Type Headache, 1990–2016: A Systematic Analysis for the Global Burden of Disease Study 2016. *Lancet Neurol.* **2018**, *17*, 954–976. [CrossRef]
11. Lempert, T.; Neuhauser, H. Epidemiology of vertigo, migraine and vestibular migraine. *J. Neurol.* **2009**, *256*, 333–338. [CrossRef] [PubMed]
12. Stolte, B.; Holle, D.; Naegel, S.; Diener, H.-C.; Obermann, M. Vestibular migraine. *Cephalalgia* **2015**, *35*, 262–270. [CrossRef] [PubMed]
13. von Brevern, M.; Neuhauser, H. Epidemiological evidence for a link between vertigo and migraine. *J. Vestib. Res.* **2011**, *21*, 299–304. [CrossRef] [PubMed]
14. Hong, S.M.; Kim, S.K.; Park, C.H.; Lee, J.H. Vestibular-evoked myogenic potentials in migrainous vertigo. *Otolaryngol. Head Neck. Surg.* **2011**, *144*, 284–287. [CrossRef] [PubMed]
15. Marcelli, V.; Piazza, F.; Pisani, F.; Marciano, E. Neuro-otological features of benign paroxysmal vertigo and benign paroxysmal positioning vertigo in children: A follow-up study. *Brain Dev.* **2006**, *28*, 80–84. [CrossRef]
16. Kayan, A.; Hood, J.D. Neuro-otological manifestations of migraine. *Brain* **1984**, *107*, 1123–1142. [CrossRef]
17. Bayazit, Y.; Yilmaz, M.; Mumbuç, S.; Kanlikama, M. Assessment of migraine-related cochleovestibular symptoms. *Rev. Laryngol. Otol. Rhinol.* **2001**, *122*, 85–88.
18. Chen, J.; Zhao, W.; Yue, X.; Zhang, P. Risk factors for the occurrence of benign paroxysmal positional vertigo: A systematic review and meta-analysis. *Front. Neurol.* **2020**, *11*, 506. [CrossRef]
19. Chen, J.; Zhang, S.; Cui, K.; Liu, C. Risk factors for benign paroxysmal positional vertigo recurrence: A systematic review and meta-analysis. *J. Neurol.* **2021**, *268*, 4117–4127. [CrossRef]
20. Ashina, M.; Katsarava, Z.; Do, T.P.; Buse, D.C.; Pozo-Rosich, P.; Özge, A.; Krymchantowski, A.V.; Lebedeva, E.R.; Ravishankar, K.; Yu, S.; et al. Migraine: Epidemiology and Systems of Care. *Lancet* **2021**, *397*, 1485–1495. [CrossRef]
21. Lee, S.H.; Kim, J.H.; Kwon, Y.S.; Lee, J.J.; Sohn, J.H. Risk of vestibulocochlear disorders in patients with migraine or non-migraine headache. *J. Pers. Med.* **2021**, *11*, 1331. [CrossRef] [PubMed]

22. Uneri, A. Migraine and benign paroxysmal positional vertigo: An outcome study of 476 patients. *Ear Nose Throat J.* **2004**, *83*, 814–815. [CrossRef] [PubMed]
23. Teixido, M.; Baker, A.; Isildak, H. Migraine and benign paroxysmal positional vertigo: A single-institution review. *J. Laryngol. Otol.* **2017**, *131*, 508–513. [CrossRef] [PubMed]
24. Chu, C.-H.; Liu, C.-J.; Lin, L.-Y.; Chen, T.-J.; Wang, S.-J. Migraine is associated with an increased risk for benign paroxysmal positional vertigo: A nationwide population-based study. *J. Headache Pain* **2015**, *16*, 62. [CrossRef] [PubMed]
25. Kim, S.K.; Hong, S.M.; Park, I.-S.; Choi, H.G. Association between migraine and benign paroxysmal positional vertigo among adults in South Korea. *JAMA Otolaryngol. Head Neck Surg.* **2019**, *145*, 307–331. [CrossRef] [PubMed]
26. Pollak, L.; Pollak, E. Headache during a cluster of benign paroxysmal positional vertigo attacks. *Ann. Otol. Rhinol. Laryngol.* **2014**, *123*, 875–880. [CrossRef]
27. Faralli, M.; Cipriani, L.; Del Zompo, M.R.; Panichi, R.; Calzolaro, L.; Ricci, G. Benign paroxysmal positional vertigo and migraine: Analysis of 186 cases. *B-ENT* **2014**, *10*, 133–139.
28. Yetiser, S.; Gokmen, M.H.A. Clinical aspects of benign paroxysmal positional vertigo associated with migraine. *Int. Tinnitus J.* **2015**, *19*, 64–68. [CrossRef]
29. Hilton, D.B.; Luryi, A.L.; Bojrab, D.I.; Babu, S.C.; Hong, R.S.; Bojrab, D.I., 2nd; Santiago Rivera, O.J.; Schutt, C.A. Comparison of associated comorbid conditions in patients with benign paroxysmal positional vertigo with or without migraine history: A large single institution study. *Am. J. Otolaryngol.* **2020**, *41*, 102650. [CrossRef]
30. Gupta, A.; Kushwaha, A.K.; Sen, K.; Bajaj, B.K. Association between benign positional vertigo and migraine in Indian population. *Indian J. Otolaryngol. Head Neck Surg.* **2022**, *74*, 420–423. [CrossRef]
31. Kim, E.K.; Pasquesi, L.; Sharon, J.D. Examining Migraine as a predictor of benign paroxysmal positional vertigo onset, severity, recurrence, and associated falls. *Cureus* **2022**, *14*, e28278. [CrossRef] [PubMed]
32. Kuritzky, A.; Ziegler, D.K.; Hassanein, R. Vertigo, motion sickness and migraine. *Headache* **1981**, *21*, 227–231. [CrossRef] [PubMed]
33. Casani, A.P.; Sellari-Franceschini, S.; Napolitano, A.; Muscatello, L.; Dallan, I. Otoneurologic dysfunctions in migraine patients with or without vertigo. *Otol. Neurotol.* **2009**, *30*, 961–967. [CrossRef] [PubMed]
34. Baloh, R.W. Neurotology of migraine. *Headache* **1997**, *37*, 615–621. [CrossRef] [PubMed]
35. Ishiyama, A.; Jacobson, K.M.; Baloh, R.W. Migraine and benign positional vertigo. *Ann. Otol. Rhinol. Laryngol.* **2000**, *109*, 377–380. [CrossRef] [PubMed]
36. El-Saied, S.; Joshua, B.-Z.; Segal, N.; Kraus, M.; Kaplan, D.M. Sudden hearing loss with simultaneous posterior semicircular canal BPPV: Possible etiology and clinical implications. *Am. J. Otolaryngol.* **2014**, *35*, 180–185. [CrossRef]
37. Jones, S.M.; Vijayakumar, S.; Dow, S.A.; Holt, J.C.; Jordan, P.M.; Luebke, A.E. Loss of α-calcitonin gene-related peptide (ACGRP) reduces otolith activation timing dynamics and impairs balance. *Front. Mol. Neurosci.* **2018**, *11*, 289. [CrossRef]
38. Kruit, M.C.; Launer, L.J.; Ferrari, M.D.; van Buchem, M.A. Infarcts in the posterior circulation territory in migraine. the population-based MRI CAMERA study. *Brain* **2005**, *128*, 2068–2077. [CrossRef]
39. Bruzzone, M.G.; Grisoli, M.; De Simone, T.; Regna-Gladin, C. Neuroradiological features of vertigo. *Neurol. Sci.* **2004**, *25* (Suppl. S1), S20–S23. [CrossRef]
40. Zhang, D.; Zhang, S.; Zhang, H.; Xu, Y.; Fu, S.; Yu, M.; Ji, P. Evaluation of vertebrobasilar artery changes in patients with benign paroxysmal positional vertigo. *Neuroreport* **2013**, *24*, 741–745. [CrossRef]
41. Lindskog, U.; Odkvist, L.; Noaksson, L.; Wallquist, J. Benign paroxysmal vertigo in childhood: A long-term follow-up. *Headache* **1999**, *39*, 33–37. [CrossRef] [PubMed]
42. Batuecas-Caletrío, A.; Martín-Sánchez, V.; Cordero-Civantos, C.; Guardado-Sánchez, L.; Marcos, M.R.; Fabián, A.H.; Benito González, J.J.; Santa Cruz-Ruiz, S. Is benign paroxysmal vertigo of childhood a migraine precursor? *Eur. J. Paediatr. Neurol.* **2013**, *17*, 397–400. [CrossRef] [PubMed]

Disclaimer/Publisher's Note: The statements, opinions and data contained in all publications are solely those of the individual author(s) and contributor(s) and not of MDPI and/or the editor(s). MDPI and/or the editor(s) disclaim responsibility for any injury to people or property resulting from any ideas, methods, instructions or products referred to in the content.

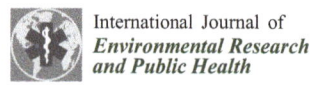

Opinion

Healthcare Professionals and Noise-Generating Tools: Challenging Assumptions about Hearing Loss Risk

Giuseppe Alberti [1], Daniele Portelli [1,2,*] and Cosimo Galletti [3]

[1] Department of Adult and Development Age Human Pathology "Gaetano Barresi", Unit of Otorhinolaryngology, University of Messina, 98125 Messina, Italy; galberti@unime.it
[2] Policlinico G. Martino, Via Consolare Valeria 1, 98125 Messina, Italy
[3] Department of Integrated Dentistry, School of Dentistry, Universitat Internacional de Catalunya, Sant Cugat del Vallès, 08017 Barcelona, Spain; cosimo88a@gmail.com
* Correspondence: danieleportelli@yahoo.it; Tel.: +39-090-2212248; Fax: +39-090-2212242

Abstract: Hearing loss is a significant global health concern, affecting billions of people and leading to various physical, mental, and social consequences. This paper focuses on the risk of noise-induced hearing loss (NIHL) among specific healthcare professionals, especially ear surgeons, orthopaedic surgeons, dentists, and dental hygienists, who frequently use noisy instruments in their professions. While studies on these professionals' noise exposure levels are limited, certain conditions and factors could pose a risk to their hearing. Measures such as engineering and administrative controls, regular audiometric testing, and the use of hearing protection devices are crucial in preventing NIHL. Early detection and intervention are also vital to mitigate further damage. This paper proposes the results of a modified screening protocol, including questionnaires, audiometry, and additional diagnostic tests to identify and address potential hearing disorders. Specific healthcare professionals should remain aware of the risks, prioritize hearing protection, and undergo regular monitoring to safeguard their long-term auditory well-being.

Keywords: noise-induced hearing loss; hidden hearing loss; ear surgeons; orthopaedic surgeons; dentists; dental hygienists; Matrix sentence test

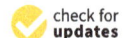

Citation: Alberti, G.; Portelli, D.; Galletti, C. Healthcare Professionals and Noise-Generating Tools: Challenging Assumptions about Hearing Loss Risk. *Int. J. Environ. Res. Public Health* **2023**, *20*, 6520. https://doi.org/10.3390/ijerph20156520

Academic Editor: Martine Hamann

Received: 10 May 2023
Revised: 20 July 2023
Accepted: 2 August 2023
Published: 4 August 2023

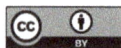

Copyright: © 2023 by the authors. Licensee MDPI, Basel, Switzerland. This article is an open access article distributed under the terms and conditions of the Creative Commons Attribution (CC BY) license (https://creativecommons.org/licenses/by/4.0/).

1. Introduction

Hearing loss affects around 1.5 billion people globally, with the World Health Organization (WHO) predicting that by 2050, the number will reach nearly 2.5 billion [1]. Hearing loss has been linked to mental illness, depression, dementia, and social isolation, and it can also impact job performance, reduce productivity, and lead to work discrimination, unemployment, or loss of income [2]. Consequently, hearing loss has become a global public health priority. The leading causes of hearing loss are ageing, noise exposure, complications during birth, genetic factors, infectious diseases, chronic ear infections, or ototoxicity [1].

Occupational noise-induced hearing loss (NIHL) is a symmetrical sensorineural hearing loss that gradually develops after continuous or intermittent noise exposure. Following exposure to loud noise, a temporary threshold shift (TTS) or temporary hearing loss is present for 16 to 48 h. During the initial stages of NIHL, pure tone audiometry may appear normal, and there may be no observable signs of hearing loss on the hearing threshold. The condition referred to as "hidden hearing loss" is characterized by the damage or loss of synaptic connections between hair cells and cochlear neurons [3].

The gradual deterioration of auditory neurons is caused by this synaptopathy, which results in abnormal speech intelligibility and involvement of the hearing threshold at high frequencies (above 3 kHz) [4,5].

According to the Occupational Safety and Health Administration (OSHA), over 20 million workers are exposed to potentially harmful noise in the workplace every year [6]. Moreover, about 18% of adults aged 20–69 who were exposed to very loud noise at work for 5 or more years reported having NIHL [7]. As a result, various occupational and environmental noise exposure standards have been established worldwide [8] (see Table 1).

Table 1. Examples of occupational noise exposure limits (adapted from: Neitzel, 2019).

Category/Limit	Allowable Exposure (dBA) for Given Time Period				
	8 h	2 h	1 h	30 min	Ceiling
European Union Directive 2003/10/EC (European Parliament and Council, 2003)					
Lower exposure action value	80	83	86	89	//
Upper exposure action value	85	88	91	94	//
Exposure limit	87	90	93	97	//
American Conference of Governmental Industrial Hygienists (ACGIH, 2018a)					
Threshold limit value	85	88	91	94	//
US National Institute for Occupational Safety and Health (NIOSH, 1998)					
Recommended exposure limit	85	88	91	94	//
U.S. Occupational Safety and Health Administration (OSHA, 1983)					
Permissible exposure limit	90	95	100	105	115
Action level	85	90	95	100	115

Note: "//", Allowable exposure dBA not provided.

The OSHA and the European Agency for Safety and Health at Work have developed a hearing conservation program for individuals exposed to a noise level of 85 dBA or higher, averaged over 8 working hours [6,9]. The A-weighting (dBA) is used to measure sound levels, accounting for the loudness perceived by the human ear, which is less sensitive to low frequencies. This program aims to raise awareness among workers about the use of protective devices to prevent NIHL [6]. However, some individuals may be more susceptible to noise exposures between 80 and 85 dB [5]. Hearing impairment has a significant impact on daily life, with limited speech understanding and impaired communication. Additionally, tinnitus, headache, dizziness, or insomnia may be associated with hearing loss. The physical and psychological stress of hearing loss can reduce productivity, and increase the risk of workplace accidents and injuries.

The International Organization for Standardization (ISO) 1999:2013, titled "Acoustics—Estimation of noise-induced hearing loss", provides comprehensive guidelines for assessing and estimating the impact of occupational noise exposure on individuals' hearing health. The key objectives of ISO 1999:2013 include establishing criteria for classifying noise-induced hearing loss, defining audiometric evaluation procedures, calculating the risk of hearing impairment, and addressing permanent noise damage. It emphasizes the importance of considering factors such as ambient noise levels and exposure duration when evaluating the risk of hearing loss. Included within the standard are tables that present examples of predicted noise-induced permanent threshold shifts (NIPTS) at frequencies of 0.5, 1, 2, 3, 4, and 6 kHz. These predictions are based on L_{EX8h} exposures of 85, 90, 95, and 100 dBA, covering exposure durations ranging from 10 to 40 years. By utilizing these tables, it becomes feasible to calculate the average estimated NIPTS for the median of a population. According to the ISO 1999 standard, hearing impairment is defined with three definitions [10]:

- An average of the hearing threshold levels at 0.5, 1, and 2 kHz that exceeds 25 dB;
- An average of the hearing threshold levels at 1, 2, and 3 kHz that exceeds 25 dB;
- An average of the hearing threshold levels at 1, 2, 3, and 4 kHz that exceeds 25 dB.

It is essential to eliminate or minimize the risk of occupational NIHL. Early detection and intervention are crucial in preventing hearing loss, which is irreversible. General prevention principles can help reduce hearing impairment, such as adopting working methods or equipment that require less exposure to noise, using shields or noise-absorbing coverings, conducting periodic audiometric testing, and utilizing hearing protectors [6].

The demanding environment of the operating room presents specific healthcare professionals with numerous challenges, and one often overlooked aspect is the potential risk of noise-induced hearing loss. In the fast-paced world of operative procedures, professionals who use noise-generating tools rely heavily on a variety of instruments to perform intricate procedures. However, the use of noisy instruments poses a unique challenge. Prolonged exposure to high levels of noise during these procedures may have detrimental effects on the professionals' hearing abilities.

This paper provides a concise overview of the hearing risks faced by some specific healthcare workers who are not considered at high risk of developing occupational NIHL.

Noise exposure levels have been recorded in various operating rooms and reported in different studies with contrasting results. The levels of noise can vary significantly depending on several factors. The design and layout of the theatres, the types of equipment and instruments utilized, as well as the procedures being performed, all contribute to the overall noise levels experienced by surgical teams [11].

Our focus is on four categories of professionals, including ear surgeons, orthopaedic surgeons, dentists, and dental hygienists, specialities that involve the use of noisy tools.

Otorhinolaryngologists, specifically ear surgeons, may face high levels of noise exposure during temporal bone drilling. Although few studies have measured the risk in the operating room, Vaisbuch et al. researched noise exposure during temporal bone drilling, even when multiple individuals were drilling simultaneously in dissection labs [4]. Some studies have reported exposure levels ranging from 68.5 to 83 dBA over an 8-h period, which did not surpass the limits established by the OSHA [12,13]. However, certain drilling conditions and environmental factors could pose a particular risk to workers' hearing. Factors such as the type of drill (air or piezoelectric), the burr type (burr diameter, cutting or diamond burr), the anatomical structure being drilled (cortical bone or mastoid cavity), and the surgical approach (translabyrinthine surgery, middle ear only, or mastoid surgery) could produce peak sound pressure levels that exceed the safe limit. Additionally, the frequency range to which the worker is exposed could vary based on these variables [4].

Orthopaedic surgeons use various power tools and loud instruments such as drills, saws, and hammers during surgery [11,14]. However, few studies have been conducted to assess noise levels in orthopaedic surgery. In a study by Goffin et al., the equivalent continuous sound pressure levels were recorded during elective arthroplasty (total hip replacement and total knee replacement), but the personal noise exposure did not reach the 80 dB daily A-weighted noise exposure level [11]. On the other hand, Mullett's study revealed that most of the cited instruments generated sound pressure levels above 90 dB, increasing the risk of premature hearing loss development. A recent study showed that noise levels reached 105.6 dBA when using a hammer and 97.9 dBA when using an oscillating saw; in these latter cases, measurements were taken considering A-weighted decibel levels, recorded with fast time weighting, once per second. [15]. However, the modernity of these tools could influence the noise level, as new instruments can generate less noise than older ones [16]. While brief and intermittent bursts of intense noises during orthopaedic surgery may reduce the risk of hearing loss or tinnitus development, further studies are necessary to confirm the association between orthopaedic occupational exposure and NIHL [11,14]. Nonetheless, personnel working in orthopaedic theatres should be aware of the potential long-term health hazard [17].

Occupational noise that may be hazardous to dental practitioners and hygienists and has been recorded even in dental healthcare settings [18–20]. Professionals in this field are exposed to noise produced by air-turbine or micromotor handpieces, ultrasonic scalers, suction tubes, and laboratory equipment. Studies have measured and reported the noise levels of these instruments, with clinical handpieces ranging from 76 to 105 dBA, suction ranging from 74 to 80 dBA, and cleaners and scalers ranging from 82 to 90 dBA [20–24]. The literature reports high variability in these noise levels, which may be influenced by various factors such as the duration of noise exposure, the type of dental speciality, and the use of faulty or worn equipment, particularly turbines [18,19]. Burk et al. have suggested that a small portion of dental professionals and students may be at risk of developing NIHL despite the reported mean 8-h time-weighted average (TWA) noise levels of 70.9 dBA [20]. Ultrasonic scalers, which produce a sound pressure level ranging from 87 to 107 dBA have also received attention as potential causes of temporary shifts in the hearing threshold, tinnitus, and a statistically significant difference in the audiometric threshold at the frequency of 3000 Hz. It should be noted, however, that these instruments generate sounds at ultra-high frequencies that are inaudible to humans regardless of intensity [25,26]. It is important to highlight that the majority of these measurements were brief recordings conducted in close proximity to operating dental instruments, rather than assessing personal exposure. Additionally, it should be noted that the A-weighting network, commonly used for occupational exposure assessments, does not fully capture noise exposures related to ultrasonic devices, as it heavily attenuates ultrasonic frequencies (>20 kHz) [20].

However, based on our experience and case series, it is not common for practitioners in these fields to utilize hearing protection devices. This lack of protection leaves them vulnerable to exposure to loud and potentially harmful levels of noise in their work environment [27].

To prevent the progression of auditory damage, early detection of these conditions is essential for individuals who are exposed to loud sounds. We firmly believe that regular audiological screening is necessary for such individuals to detect a hearing impairment.

Below, we outline a modified adult screening procedure recommended by the World Health Organization, which is followed at our tertiary referral centre, Policlinico "G. Martino" in Messina (Italy) [28] (see Figure 1). Due to the lack of validation of our screening protocol, the full substantiation of its effectiveness remains inconclusive. However, it may hold potential as a valuable tool in clinical practice, aiding in early identification of potential hearing issues for timely intervention and improved patient outcomes. Furthermore, we present a retrospective analysis of data from the past 2 years, obtained from 42 people who underwent screening.

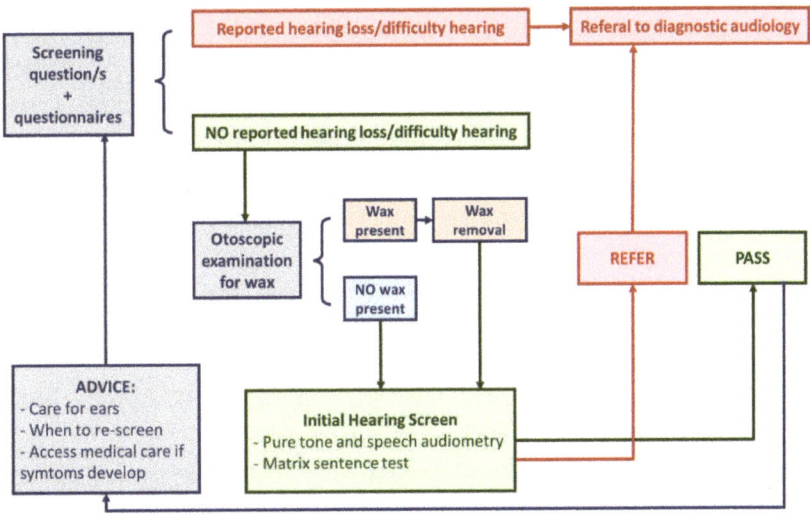

Figure 1. Modified WHO adult hearing screening (Adapted from: Hearing screening. Consideration for implementation. WHO. 2021 [28]).

2. Materials and Methods

2.1. Participants

A total of 42 individuals, comprising ear surgeons (10 subjects), orthopaedic surgeons (14 subjects), dentists, and dental hygienists (18 subjects), underwent a hearing screening (see Figure 1). These participants were selected based on specific inclusion criteria, which included a minimum of 10 years of occupational experience in their respective fields and consistent exposure to noise-emitting tools during this period. All subjects did not use any type of noise attenuator or hearing protector. They also had no pre-existing diagnosed conditions or were not on chronic medication therapies for any specific medical conditions. Subjects were invited to undergo free hearing screening through online advertisements, word-of-mouth among acquaintances, or direct invitations. All tests were conducted at Policlinico "G. Martino" in Messina, a tertiary referral centre. The data presented here are reflective of the past two years.

2.2. Screening Questions and Questionnaires

Simple anamnestic questions regarding hearing are employed as part of the screening process. These questions provide a comprehensive overview of the individual's hearing health and help direct the screening investigation. A combination of binary (Yes/No) response questions and scored questions are utilized (see Table 2).

Table 2. Examples of questions and questionnaires for screening (Adapted from Hearing screening. Consideration for implementation. WHO. 2021 [28]).

Screening Questions and Questionnaires
A. Yes/No questions:
a. Do you have any hearing problem now?
b. Do you have a diagnosed hearing loss?
c. Do you use hearing aids?
d. Have you noticed any changes in your hearing abilities recently?
e. Do you experience difficulty understanding conversations in noisy environments?
f. Have you ever had any exposure to loud noise, either in your personal or professional life?
g. Have you ever experienced ringing or buzzing sounds in your ears (tinnitus)?
h. Are there any instances where you struggle to hear certain frequencies or sounds?
i. Have you ever had your hearing tested or undergone any auditory assessments?
j. Are you aware of the risks associated with noise-induced hearing loss?
k. Have you noticed any impact on your hearing after performing the procedures or being in the operating room?
B. Scaled questions:
a. How would you characterize your hearing?
i. Excellent
ii. Very good
iii. Good
iv. Fair
v. Poor
C. Existing screening questionnaire
a. Self-Efficacy for Situational Communication Management Questionnaire (SESMQ)
b. Noise Exposure Questionnaire (NEQ) and 1-min Noise Screen
c. Hearing Handicap Inventory for the Elderly (HHIE)

These questions allow for quick assessments and are designed to capture specific aspects of the individual's hearing health. They cover topics such as exposure to loud noise, history of ear infections or trauma, and the use of hearing protection devices. These questions enable healthcare professionals to identify potential risk factors and determine the need for further evaluation.

Furthermore, validated questionnaires can be employed to delve deeper into the initial investigation. These questionnaires have been extensively tested and proven to be reliable tools for assessing specific aspects of hearing. By utilizing these validated questionnaires, healthcare professionals can gather more comprehensive data and gain further insights into the individual's hearing health status.

Typically, we employ three questionnaires:

1. The Self-Efficacy for Situational Communication Management Questionnaire (SESMQ), which measures the perceived self-efficacy for managing communication in individuals with hearing loss. The SESMQ questionnaire consists of 20 questions, each divided into two scales, and the subject is required to respond by assigning a score from 1 to 10. The first scale assesses hearing ability (SESMQH), while the second scale evaluates the level of confidence (SESMQ). Each subscale has a score ranging from 10 to 200. The total score is the sum of the two subscale scores [29];

2. The Noise Exposure Questionnaire (NEQ), which quantifies personal annual noise exposure from both occupational and non-occupational sources. The NEQ questionnaire consists of three sections: the first section includes demographic information, the second section contains six screening questions that assess exposure to high levels of noise, and the third section consists of eleven questions related to participation in noisy activities, on which the annual exposure level is calculated. Three questions in the second section (1-min Noise Screen) serve as a screening tool to assess exposure to high levels of noise, with a score greater than 4 indicating a high risk of developing NIHL (Noise-Induced Hearing Loss). The NEQ questionnaire calculates the annual noise exposure, and the risk of developing NIHL occurs when the $L_{Aeq8760h}$ (annual equivalent sound level) is equal to or greater than 79 dB [30];

3. The Hearing Handicap Inventory for the Elderly (HHIE), which assesses the impact of hearing impairment on emotional and social adjustment. The HHIE questionnaire consists of 25 questions. The individual assigns a score ranging from "yes" (4 points), "sometimes" (2 points), to "no" (0 points). The total score ranges from 0 to 100 [31].

2.3. Audiological Screening Tests

Pure-tone audiometry, speech audiometry, and the free-field Matrix sentence test are used as audiological screening tests. These are conducted within a soundproof booth that attenuated environmental noise by 40 dB SPL. The tests are performed using the Madsen Astera2 audiometer (Otosuite V. 8.84.0 software, Taastrup, Denmark), which had been calibrated within the last 12 months prior to the measurements. For the audiometric evaluations, TDH39 earphones, a B71 bone vibrator, and speakers are utilized.

Pure-tone audiometry is employed to determine the individual's hearing threshold. Speech audiometry is also conducted using spondaic disyllabic Italian words [32]. The word recognition score (WRS) is measured as the percentage of correctly recognized words when a list of ten words is presented to the individual. No masking noise is used during this test. The air conduction pure-tone average (AC PTA) and the bone conduction pure-tone average (BC PTA) are automatically computed based on the hearing thresholds at 500, 1000, and 2000 Hz; furthermore, a modified air conduction pure-tone average (AC mPTA) and a modified bone conduction pure-tone average (BC mPTA) considering the frequencies 1000, 2000, and 4000 Hz are utilized, as suggested by Moore et al., to better assess noise-induced hearing loss. This modified PTA approach allows for a more focused evaluation of the specific frequency range commonly affected by noise-induced hearing impairments [33].

To assess speech-in-noise intelligibility, the Italian Matrix sentence test is performed. For this test, two speakers are positioned at a distance of 1 m from the participant, with one on the left side and the other on the right side (azimuth angles of −45° and +45°, respectively). This is an adaptive speech-in-noise test that consists of 20 randomly generated sentences, each composed of five words, with a background noise interfering with the speech message. The subject is asked to repeat each word they can hear [34]. If the subject accurately repeats at least three words, the speech level is decreased; otherwise, it is increased. The Matrix software computes the speech reception threshold (SRT), which represents the 50% threshold of speech intelligibility in noise (dB SNR). This test is valuable for evaluating both the individual's ability to recognize speech in noisy environments and the effectiveness of hearing aids [35,36].

The purpose of the audiological screening tests is to detect the possible presence of noise-induced hearing loss or other disorders in the auditory system such as tinnitus or abnormal speech intelligibility. Noise-induced hearing loss (NIHL) is a symmetrical sensorineural hearing loss that gradually develops after continuous or intermittent noise exposure [5].

2.4. Procedure

All subjects underwent an anamnestic questionnaire (see Table 2) to assess their hearing health status. These questions were designed to guide subsequent screening steps. All subjects were administered the SESMQ questionnaire and the 1-min Noise Screen questionnaire. It should be noted that the SESMQ questionnaire was initially developed for elderly subjects with acquired hearing loss, and its validity in younger individuals has not yet been established [29]. However, this questionnaire can provide an estimate of the subjectively perceived level of disability in communication ability. A score of 5 or higher on the 1-min Noise Screen indicates a high risk of noise exposure, and thus, these subjects were further evaluated with the comprehensive NEQ questionnaire. Subjects who perceived a decrease in their hearing abilities or tinnitus were also administered the HHIE questionnaire.

When questionable results were obtained, an audiological assessment was strongly recommended. For individuals who do not report hearing problems, a second screening test was performed.

Subsequently, all subjects underwent otomicroscopic examination to assess the presence of earwax, which was removed if necessary. Following this, pure-tone audiometry, speech audiometry with headphones, and the free-field Matrix Sentence Test were performed.

"PASS" indicates a condition in which there is no alteration in the audiometric threshold or speech-in-noise intelligibility, as determined by the results of the Matrix sentence test. On the other hand, "REFER" indicates an alteration in one or both of the audiologic tests used.

Individuals who receive a "PASS" result in these hearing screening tests will undergo another screening after about two years. Those who receive a "REFER" result will require further evaluation for the presence of any "red flags" alerts, such as rapidly progressive hearing loss, unilateral hearing loss, ear pain, ear discharge, dizziness, or previous diagnosis of ear disease [28].

Doubtful results in these screening tests required more accurate diagnostic approaches, such as auditory brainstem response (ABR), otoacoustic emissions (OAE), magnetic resonance imaging (MRI) of the brain and brainstem, and computed tomography (CT), tympanometry and acoustic reflex testing, etc. Furthermore, overlapping pathological conditions may be present in the patients, and they should not be underestimated.

Results

In our case series, a total of 42 subjects (27 males and 15 females) underwent screening. Among them, 10 were ear surgeons, 14 were orthopaedic surgeons, and 18 were dentists or dental hygienists. The average age of these subjects was 48.5 ± 9.5 years, with an average work experience of 22.1 ± 9.5 years (see Table 3).

Analysing the data obtained from the audiometric thresholds, the mean of AC mPTA for the right ear was 19.2 ± 7.6 dB HL, and for the left ear, it was 19.4 ± 7.2 dB HL. As for the word recognition score (WRS), all subjects achieved the 100% intelligibility threshold.

Table 3. Study population. N, number; %, percentage; M, mean; SD, standard deviation; AC PTA, air conduction pure tone average; AC mPTA, air conduction modified pure tone average; BC PTA, bone conduction pure tone average; BC mPTA, bone conduction modified pure tone average; WRS, word recognition score; SRT, speech reception threshold; SNR, signal to noise ratio.

	N (%); M ± SD
Gender	42 (100%)
Male	27 (64%)
Female	15 (36%)
Profession	42 (100%)
Ear surgeons	10 (24%)
Orthopaedic surgeons	14 (33%)
Dentists and dental hygienists	18 (43%)
Age (years)	48.5 ± 9.5
Worked years (years)	22 ± 9.5
AC PTA Right (dB HL)	17.1 ± 5.5
AC mPTA Right (dB HL)	19.2 ± 7.6
AC PTA Left (dB HL)	18.0 ± 5.5
AC mPTA Left (dB HL)	19.4 ± 7.2
BC PTA Right (dB HL)	11.9 ± 5.2
BC mPTA Right (dB HL)	14.0 ± 7.5
BC PTA Left (dB HL)	12.6 ± 4.7
BC mPTA Left (dB HL)	14.0 ± 6.8
WRS Right % (dB HL)	100 ± 0 (40.7 ± 7.1)
WRS Left % (dB HL)	100 ± 0 (40.7 ± 7.1)
SRT (dB SNR)	−6.2 ± 0.9

Regarding the speech reception threshold (SRT), the average was −6.3 ± 0.9 dB SNR. Two subjects recorded an increased SRT despite having a normal hearing threshold (−3.6 dB SNR, −4.8 dB SNR). These values contradicted the normative data presented by Puglisi et al. for the Italian version of the Matrix sentence test [34].

The subjects were then stratified into two groups based on the presence or absence of a hearing handicap. A "hearing handicap" is defined as an impairment in the auditory system that can be objectively measured through the used screening audiological tests or subjectively reported by the person from the anamnestic questions and questionnaires for screening, such as tinnitus or decreased speech-in-noise intelligibility. Thirteen subjects showed evidence of hearing issues: high-frequency notch at 4 kHz (four subjects), otosclerosis (one subject), high-frequency hearing loss (three subjects), tinnitus (three subjects), and elevated SRT with normal hearing threshold (two subjects) (see Tables 4 and 5).

From the screening anamnestic questions (questions "j" and "k", see Table 2), it was observed that all subjects lacked awareness of the noise they were exposed to, considering it insufficiently intense to cause noise-induced hearing loss. Additionally, from a subjective perspective, four subjects without a hearing handicap and three subjects with a hearing handicap reported experiencing a sensation of muffled hearing immediately following the cessation of exposure to the noisy instrument. All subjects reported that this sensation lasted between 5 and 15 s and disappeared thereafter. We hypothesize that this phenomenon may be attributed to temporary auditory fatigue.

Table 4. Number of subjects with and without hearing handicap. N, number; %, percentage; SRT, speech reception threshold.

Subjects with	N (%)
No hearing handicap	29 (69%)
Hearing handicap	
4 kHz notch on hearing threshold	4 (9.5%)
Otosclerosis	1 (2.4%)
High frequencies hearing loss	3 (7.1%)
Tinnitus	3 (7.1%)
Increased SRT with normal hearing threshold	2 (4.8%)

Table 5. Subjects' data obtained from audiological screening tests. M, mean; SD, standard deviation AC PTA, air conduction pure tone average; AC mPTA, air conduction modified pure tone average; SRT, speech reception threshold.

Subjects with	AC PTA (Right; Left) (M ± SD)	AC mPTA (Right; Left) (M ± SD)	SRT (M ± SD)
No hearing handicap	14.6 ± 3.2; 15.7 ± 2.6	15.3 ± 3; 15.8 ± 2.4	−6.7 ± 0.5
Hearing handicap			
4 kHz notch on hearing threshold	21.3 ± 3.5; 20.5 ± 5.8	29.3 ± 2.9; 27.3 ± 4.3	−5.2 ± 0.4
Otosclerosis	25; 35 *	23; 32 *	−5.2 *
High frequencies hearing loss	29.7 ± 2.5; 30 ± 2;	38.7 ± 2.9; 38.3 ± 2.9	−5.4 ± 0.3
Tinnitus	21.3 ± 5.1; 20.7 ± 3.2	23.3 ± 4.2; 22.3 ± 0.6	−5.6 ± 0.2
Increased SRT with normal hearing threshold	17.0 ± 0; 16.5 ± 2.1	17.5 ± 0.7; 17.5 ± 0.7	−4.2 ± 0.8

* The AC PTA, the AC mPTA, and the SRT pertain to a single case only; data are presented as mean.

The average total score of the SESMQ questionnaire was 326.2 ± 32.4. The questionnaire revealed lower scores in subjects with hearing problems (see Table 6).

Table 6. SESMQ questionnaire results. M, mean; SD, standard deviation; SESMQH, Self-Efficacy for Situational Communication Management Questionnaire Hearing ability score; SESMQC, Self-Efficacy for Situational Communication Management Questionnaire Confidence score; SESMQ, Self-Efficacy for Situational Communication Management Questionnaire global score.

Subjects with (N)	SESMQH (M ± SD)	SESMQC (M ± SD)	SESMQ (M ± SD)
No hearing handicap (29)	175.9 ± 5.3	166.0 ± 6.2	341.9 ± 10.9
Hearing handicap (13)	148.2 ± 17.9	142.9 ± 19.9	291.1 ± 37.2
Total of subjects (42)	167.4 ± 16.8	158.8 ± 16.1	326.2 ± 32.4

On the other hand, the 1-min Noise Screen allowed the identification of individuals at higher risk of developing noise-induced hearing loss, considering both recreational and job activities. The average score obtained was 3.3 ± 1.4, indicating that these subjects were not at a high risk of noise-induced hearing loss (see Table 7). It should be noted that this is the average score among all participants. However, out of the 42 participants, 8 obtained scores higher than 4, and thus, they underwent the complete NEQ questionnaire. Only two of them demonstrated annual $L_{Aeq8760h}$ (annual equivalent sound level) exposure levels exceeding 79 dB, indicating a risk of developing hearing loss.

Table 7. 1-min Noise Screen results. M, mean; SD, standard deviation.

Subjects with	1 min Noise Screen (M ± SD)
No hearing handicap	3.0 ± 1.3
Hearing handicap	4.1 ± 1.3
Total of subjects	3.3 ± 1.4

Regarding the HHIE questionnaire, the test was administered to the 13 subjects who reported a hearing handicap; the average score was 17.4 ± 11. Only subjects who had a hearing handicap were administered this test; no other subjects reported any hearing problems.

We want to clarify that no statistical analysis has been conducted as the presented article takes the form of an "opinion" rather than a research study aimed at demonstrating the association between the use of noise-emitting tools and noise-induced hearing loss or even other hearing disorders. The screening protocol is currently undergoing validation, and the results presented are only preliminary data. Subjects were stratified solely for descriptive purposes and not for comparison. The literature contains variable data regarding exposure levels, making it unable to definitively state the absence of a real risk for these individuals. Therefore, the possibility of developing noise-induced hearing loss or other auditory issues should always be taken into consideration.

3. Discussion

The best way to reduce the risk of developing occupational NIHL is through prevention measures, as the condition is irreversible and there are currently no effective treatments available. The prevention program is based on three levels: primary prevention, which involves reducing noise exposure levels below hazardous levels; secondary prevention, which focuses on early detection of hearing loss to prevent further damage; and tertiary prevention, which aims to reduce disability or handicap when significant impairment is already present [9,37].

The European Agency for Safety and Health at Work emphasizes the importance of maintaining a safe and healthy work environment, including periodic monitoring of noise exposure. When high levels of noise are detected, engineering and administrative controls are necessary to prevent irreversible damage to the inner ear. These controls include: (1) selecting appropriate work equipment; (2) providing adequate information and training to ensure proper use of work equipment; (3) reducing noise levels through technical means; (4) implementing maintenance programs for work equipment, workplace, and workplace systems; (5) organizing work to minimize noise levels; (6) limiting the duration and intensity of noise exposure; (7) establishing work schedules that include adequate rest periods [9].

The risk of developing occupational NIHL can be significantly reduced or eliminated when the noise level is kept below 80 dBA. Legal standards for noise levels have been established by various countries [8]. When noise levels cannot be reduced, workers should use hearing protection devices. Two types of hearing protection devices are currently available: active and passive devices. Research has demonstrated that these devices are effective at reducing sound levels, allowing workers to locate the source of sounds, and enabling communication [38].

Elevated noise levels have been observed to have a detrimental impact on patient outcomes and impair the performance of healthcare professionals in the operating room. Despite the increase in decibel levels caused by playing music in the operating room, the majority of surveyed staff expressed a positive inclination towards having music during surgery, believing it to enhance both individual and team performance. Overall, music was not perceived as a distraction or hindrance to communication [39]. Some studies indicated a notable decrease in postoperative complication rates when noise levels were reduced during surgery [40–42]. In a study conducted in a paediatric surgery department, various measures were implemented to reduce noise levels, including the use of sound-reduction devices, behavioural guidelines restricting conversation, minimizing the opening of operating room doors, and managing monitor alarms. This comprehensive noise reduction program resulted in a significant reduction of approximately 50% in decibel levels during paediatric surgical procedures [42].

Other measures of well-being could be applied in the environments where operative procedures are conducted. In a study that proposed the revitalization of a park, it was highlighted that it is not only necessary to reduce noise exposure levels or introduce positive sounds, but also to implement measures that enhance overall well-being. A similar approach could be employed in the workplaces where the subjects under consideration operate. Further investigation is needed to explore the most effective measures, making this area a promising research field yet to be fully explored [43].

Secondary prevention is achieved through regular audiometric testing. Implementing regular auditory assessments and monitoring programs can help detect any early signs of hearing loss in professionals who use noise-generating tools. Prompt identification of hearing impairment allows for timely intervention and the implementation of strategies to mitigate further damage.

However, there is still some uncertainty in the literature regarding noise exposure for these subjects who work with noisy instruments. Although these workers are not typically considered at high risk for developing occupational NIHL, it has been reported that noises below the action level can cause temporary and potentially long-term hearing damage [4].

Animal studies have shown that moderate noise exposure (100 dB SPL for 2 h) can cause a TTS without resulting in hair cell loss. However, repeated TTSs, even with threshold recovery, can alter cochlear responses to suprathreshold sound levels. This can result in a synaptopathy, which is characterized by a reduced number of auditory nerve fibres' activation and a decrease in their firing rate or synchrony. This condition is known as "hidden hearing loss" and is characterized by a normal hearing threshold but difficulties in complex listening tasks, such as word recognition, accurate speech, and sound detection in noisy environments [44].

According to Moore et al., pure tone and speech audiometry are valuable tests in diagnosing NIHL. NIHL caused by different types of noises can be distinguished. Additionally, it is advisable to compare the patient's hearing threshold with the age-related hearing levels for a non-noise-exposed population, typically using the 50th percentile as specified in ISO 7029 (2017). The NIHL should be quantified for each ear by considering the mean hearing threshold across the frequencies of 1, 2, and 4 kHz [33].

The diagnosis of hidden hearing loss warrants a separate discussion. Kohrman et al. have described three diagnostic approaches for this. The first approach involves the auditory brainstem response (ABR), which shows a reduction in the amplitude of the ABR I peak without any changes in ABR threshold or latency. This reduction correlates with the degree of cochlear synaptopathy. The second approach involves frequency following responses (FFRs), which demonstrate a decline in modulation frequency near 1 kHz, correlating with synaptic loss. The third approach involves a weaker middle ear muscle reflex response in individuals with hidden hearing loss [44].

In this study, we presented the data related to the screening protocol followed at our tertiary referral centre. It is important to note that these are preliminary findings. The screening program has been ongoing for two years, and concrete data on subject follow-up are not yet available.

As mentioned earlier, the subjects were recruited among ear surgeons, orthopaedic surgeons, dentists, and dental hygienists. We deemed it appropriate to select only subjects with more than 10 years of experience, as the risk of noise-induced hearing loss increases with prolonged exposure.

As outlined in the Materials and Methods section, the initial step involved collecting subject histories to guide the clinician in the appropriate screening pathway. The SESMQ questionnaire and the 1-min Noise Screen were administered to all subjects, while the HHIE questionnaire was given only to those who reported subjective hearing loss or a hearing handicap. It is important to note that these questionnaires are easy and reliable tools for initial diagnostic assessment but should be integrated with objective tests. Questionnaires provide subjective estimates in a rapid manner, as they can be completed in a few minutes. They also have the advantage of being sent via email or filled in online, allowing for quick data collection and early identification of individuals at risk of hearing loss. However, it should be noted that the 1-min Noise Screen may not identify subjects at risk of noise-induced hearing loss since these people may not perceive their noise exposure as risky. This may necessitate the administration of the full NEQ questionnaire.

Regarding the administration of the HHIE questionnaire, in our protocol, it is given only to subjects who perceive hearing loss. In this case, as well, biases may occur as some subjects may perceive hearing loss despite having normal auditory function (not in our case series).

Furthermore, questionnaires are tools that should be used to rapidly obtain an effective estimation of the risk of noise-induced hearing loss or deafness. Therefore, a streamlined procedure must be applied when extending the screening protocol to many subjects to ensure compliance.

However, in our protocol, all subjects subsequently undergo more reliable tests such as pure-tone audiometry, speech audiometry, and the Matrix sentence test. Subjects with normal results, indicating a PASS, are rescreened after 2 years. Those with hearing problems undergo more comprehensive examinations.

In our case series of 42 subjects, 13 individuals demonstrated a hearing handicap: these were referred for further instrumental examinations. The data for these patients are currently unavailable as the diagnostic assessment is still ongoing; hence, concrete results cannot be presented at this time.

Out of the eight subjects who completed the full NEQ questionnaire, only two subjects exceeded an annual $L_{Aeq8760h}$ of 79 dB: one subject with a notch at 4 kHz and one subject without hearing impairment.

It is important to reiterate that the data presented in this study are preliminary. The hearing problems observed in these subjects cannot be definitively attributed to noise-induced damage: modifiable risk factors (smoking, alcohol, obesity, etc.) and non-modifiable factors (age, sex, genetics), as well as comorbidities or ototoxic drugs, can influence the possibility of hearing damage. The purpose of this study is not to establish a causal relationship between the "risk factor" of using noise-emitting tools and the "disease" itself, namely noise-induced hearing loss, but rather to raise awareness about the potential impact of the work environments and tools utilized on the individuals' auditory system. Establishing a potential correlation between noise-induced hearing loss in the considered healthcare workers requires appropriate studies. The noise exposure levels to which the subjects are exposed, necessary according to the ISO 1999–2013 standard to assess the risk of developing noise-induced hearing loss, were not considered in this paper, as the focus is to describe a possible streamlined and rapid screening program. Subjects may be exposed to varying levels of noise, and it is uncertain whether some of these levels are of sufficient intensity to cause auditory damage. Measuring exposure levels requires specific protocols that are challenging to implement in a screening program. However, the purpose of this analysis is to draw attention to a relevant public health issue. We are convinced that the conflicting results present in the literature require further confirmation to avoid underestimating the risk faced by these individuals and to identify the most appropriate screening protocol. Due to the presence of numerous limitations and biases in our work, as a future perspective, and an expansion of the scientific literature, a more refined and validated screening program should be developed. Studies demonstrating the association between noise-emitting operative tools and noise-induced hearing loss, or other hearing impairments, should be conducted, considering the execution of randomized clinical trials with a larger sample size or multicenter studies. Additionally, evaluating noise exposure levels and taking into account human exposure to noise, considering the position of the operator's head and body, would provide more accurate measurements. Therefore, a binaural measurement approach would be recommended.

4. Conclusions

Noise-induced hearing loss is a real occupational hazard faced by surgeons and other healthcare professionals due to prolonged exposure to high levels of noise in the operating room. Preventing occupational noise-induced hearing loss is crucial as the condition is irreversible and currently has no cure. To achieve this goal, a prevention program is recommended.

Creating awareness among professionals who use noise-generating tools about the importance of noise management in the operating room is essential. Education and training programs can emphasize the significance of adopting noise reduction strategies while using these instruments when necessary.

Despite being exposed to high noise levels, these subjects may not be considered a high-risk group for developing hearing handicaps. Factors such as the short duration of exposure, distance from noise sources, awareness of the risks, and regular auditory assessments contribute to the preservation of their hearing health.

The variability in noise levels underscores the importance of conducting individualized assessments for each operating room. Understanding the specific factors that contribute to noise generation in each specialty can aid in implementing appropriate noise control measures.

From the data we collected, out of the 42 subjects analysed, 13 individuals had a hearing handicap. Among these, one case was attributed to otosclerosis and not related to noise exposure. As for the remaining 12 subjects, it cannot be definitively stated that their hearing handicap is solely attributable to noise exposure, but it cannot be ruled out either. These individuals exhibit deficits compatible with noise-induced damage. While we acknowledge that our screening currently lacks validation, the analysis of data from these subjects still revealed the presence of some individuals with a hearing handicap.

In this article, we aim to advocate for the importance of regular screenings in these individuals, as there is a lack of awareness, based on our experience, regarding the potential risk of developing hearing impairment. Although the association has not been proven, screening can serve as an early diagnostic tool for identifying potential hearing deficits among these subjects.

If a potential association between noise-induced hearing loss and healthcare workers who use noisy instruments is confirmed, efforts should be directed towards optimizing the acoustic environment in operating rooms through the use of sound-absorbing materials, proper room design, and the adoption of quieter surgical instruments where feasible. Additionally, the use of personal protective equipment, such as noise attenuators or hearing protectors, should be considered to minimize the risk of prolonged exposure to high noise levels.

We believe that further research and collaboration between healthcare professionals, audiologists, and equipment manufacturers are needed to establish standardized guidelines and best practices for noise control in operating rooms. By addressing the variability in noise levels across different specialties and implementing appropriate mitigation strategies, the overall work environment can be made safer and more conducive to optimal surgical outcomes and the well-being of surgical teams.

However, it is crucial for these workers to remain vigilant, prioritize hearing protection, and continue to monitor their hearing to ensure long-term auditory well-being, protecting the "gift of sound".

Author Contributions: Conceptualization, G.A., D.P. and C.G.; methodology, G.A. and D.P.; formal analysis, D.P.; investigation, G.A. and C.G.; data curation, G.A.; writing—original draft preparation, D.P.; writing—review and editing, D.P. and C.G.; visualization, G.A. and C.G.; supervision, C.G.

project administration, G.A. and C.G. All authors have read and agreed to the published version of the manuscript.

Funding: This research received no external funding.

Institutional Review Board Statement: The study was conducted in accordance with the Declaration of Helsinki, the results presented in this paper represent a retrospective analysis of data obtained from our screening protocol. Furthermore, the data presented in this paper do not violate the privacy of the subjects. As this screening campaign was conducted for awareness purposes rather than research, no ethical committee approval was sought; all subjects voluntarily chose to undergo the tests; all the tests involved in this screening were non-invasive and posed no risk for the participants.

Informed Consent Statement: Informed consent was obtained from all involved subjects for the execution of the screening protocol and the use of personal data.

Data Availability Statement: The data presented in this study are available on request to the corresponding author. The data are not publicly available as they may contain sensitive patient information, including medical history, questionnaire results (which may include personal information), and audiological test results.

Conflicts of Interest: The authors declare no conflict of interest.

References

1. World Health Organization. *World Report on Hearing*; World Health Organization: Geneva, Switzerland, 2021.
2. Dritsakis, G.; Trenkova, L.; Śliwińska-Kowalska, M.; Brdarić, D.; Pontoppidan, N.H.; Katrakazas, P.; Bamiou, D.E. Public health policy-making for hearing loss: Stakeholders' evaluation of a novel eHealth tool. *Health Res. Policy Syst.* **2020**, *18*, 125. [CrossRef] [PubMed]
3. Plack, C.J.; Barker, D.; Prendergast, G. Perceptual consequences of "hidden" hearing loss. *Trends Hear.* **2014**, *18*, 2331216514550621. [CrossRef] [PubMed]
4. Vaisbuch, Y.; Alyono, J.C.; Kandathil, C.; Wu, S.H.; Fitzgerald, M.B.; Jackler, R.K. Occupational Noise Exposure and Risk for Noise-Induced Hearing Loss Due to Temporal Bone Drilling. *Otol. Neurotol.* **2018**, *39*, 693–699. [CrossRef] [PubMed]
5. Mirza, R.; Kirchner, D.B.; Dobie, R.A.; Crawford, J. ACOEM Task Force on Occupational Hearing Loss. *J. Occup. Environ. Med.* **2018**, *60*, e498–e501. [CrossRef]
6. Occupational Noise Exposure. Available online: https://www.osha.gov/noise (accessed on 6 May 2023).
7. Hoffman, H.J.; Dobie, R.A.; Losonczy, K.G.; Themann, C.L.; Flamme, G.A. Declining Prevalence of Hearing Loss in US Adults Aged 20 to 69 Years. *JAMA Otolaryngol. Head Neck Surg.* **2017**, *143*, 274–285. [CrossRef]
8. Neitzel, R.L.; Fligor, B.J. Risk of noise-induced hearing loss due to recreational sound: Review and recommendations. *J. Acoust. Soc. Am.* **2019**, *146*, 3911. [CrossRef]
9. Directive 2003/10/EC of the European Parliament and of the Council of 6 February 2003. Available online: https://eur-lex.europa.eu/legal-content/EN/TXT/?uri=CELEX:02003L0010-20190726 (accessed on 6 May 2023).
10. *ISO 1999-2013*; Acoustics—Estimation of Noise-Induced Hearing Loss. ISO: Geneva, Switzerland, 2013.
11. Goffin, J.S.O.; MacDonald, D.R.W.; Neilly, D.; Munro, C.; Ashcroft, G.P. Evaluation of sound levels in elective orthopaedic theatres during primary hip and knee arthroplasty. *Surgeon* **2022**, *20*, 225–230. [CrossRef]
12. Lee, H.K.; Lee, E.H.; Choi, J.Y.; Choi, H.S.; Kim, H.N. Noise level of drilling instruments during mastoidectomy. *Yonsei Med. J.* **1999**, *40*, 339–342. [CrossRef]
13. Verhaert, N.; Moyaert, N.; Godderis, L.; Debruyne, F.; Desloovere, C.; Luts, H. Noise exposure of care providers during otosurgical procedures. *B-ENT* **2013**, *9*, 3–8.
14. Ullah, R.; Bailie, N.; Crowther, S.; Cullen, J. Noise exposure in orthopaedic practice: Potential health risk. *J. Laryngol. Otol.* **2004**, *118*, 413–416. [CrossRef]
15. Simpson, J.P.; Hamer, A.J. How noisy are total knee and hip replacements? *J. Perioper. Pract.* **2017**, *27*, 292–295. [CrossRef]
16. Mullett, H.; Synnott, K.; Quinlan, W. Occupational noise levels in orthopaedic surgery. *Ir. J. Med. Sci.* **1999**, *168*, 106. [CrossRef] [PubMed]
17. Hawi, N.; Alazzawi, S.; Schmitz, A.; Kreibich, T.; Gehrke, T.; Kendoff, D.; Haasper, C. Noise levels during total hip arthroplasty: The silent health hazard. *Hip Int.* **2020**, *30*, 679–683. [CrossRef] [PubMed]
18. Messano, G.A.; Petti, S. General dental practitioners and hearing impairment. *J. Dent.* **2012**, *40*, 821–828. [CrossRef] [PubMed]
19. Henneberry, K.; Hilland, S.; Haslam, S.K. Are dental hygienists at risk for noise-induced hearing loss? A literature review. *Can. J. Dent. Hyg.* **2021**, *55*, 110–119.
20. Burk, A.; Neitzel, R.L. An exploratory study of noise exposures in educational and private dental clinics. *J. Occup. Environ. Hyg.* **2016**, *13*, 741–749. [CrossRef]
21. Kilpatrick, H.C. Decibel ratings of dental office sounds. *J. Prosthet. Dent.* **1981**, *45*, 175–178. [CrossRef]

22. Setcos, J.C.; Mahyuddin, A. Noise levels encountered in dental clinical and laboratory practice. *Int. J. Prosthodont.* **1998**, *11*, 150–157.
23. Sampaio Fernandes, J.C.; Carvalho, A.P.; Gallas, M.; Vaz, P.; Matos, P.A. Noise levels in dental schools. *Eur. J. Dent. Educ.* **2006**, *10*, 32–37. [CrossRef]
24. Kadanakuppe, S.; Bhat, P.K.; Jyothi, C.; Ramegowda, C. Assessment of noise levels of the equipments used in the dental teaching institution, Bangalore. *Indian J. Dent. Res.* **2011**, *22*, 424–431. [CrossRef]
25. Wilson, J.D.; Darby, M.L.; Tolle, S.L.; Sever, J.C., Jr. Effects of occupational ultrasonic noise exposure on hearing of dental hygienists: A pilot study. *J. Dent. Hyg.* **2002**, *76*, 262–269. [PubMed]
26. Arabaci, T.; Çiçek, Y.; Canakçi, C.F. Sonic and ultrasonic scalers in periodontal treatment: A review. *Int. J. Dent. Hyg.* **2007**, *5*, 2–12. [CrossRef] [PubMed]
27. Prasad, K.R.; Reddy, K.T. Live recordings of sound levels during the use of powered instruments in ENT surgery. *J. Laryngol. Otol.* **2003**, *117*, 532–535. [CrossRef]
28. World Health Organization. *Hearing Screening: Consideration for Implementation*; World Health Organization: Geneva, Switzerland, 2021.
29. Jennings, M.B.; Cheesman, M.F.; Laplante-Lévesque, A. Psychometric properties of the self-efficacy for situational communication management questionnaire (SESMQ). *Ear Hear.* **2014**, *35*, 221–229. [CrossRef] [PubMed]
30. Johnson, T.A.; Cooper, S.; Stamper, G.C.; Chertoff, M. Noise Exposure Questionnaire: A Tool for Quantifying Annual Noise Exposure. *J. Am. Acad. Audiol.* **2017**, *28*, 14–35. [CrossRef]
31. Ventry, I.M.; Weinstein, B.E. The hearing handicap inventory for the elderly: A new tool. *Ear Hear.* **1982**, *3*, 128–134. [CrossRef]
32. Turrini, M.; Cutugno, F.; Maturi, P.; Prosser, S.; Leoni, F.A.; Arslan, E. Nuove parole bisillabiche per audiometriavocale in lingua Italiana [Bisyllabic words for speech audiometry: A new Italian material]. *Acta Otorhinolaryngol. Ital.* **1993**, *13*, 63–77.
33. Moore, B.C.J.; Lowe, D.A.; Cox, G. Guidelines for Diagnosing and Quantifying Noise-Induced Hearing Loss. *Trends Hear.* **2022**, *26*, 23312165221093156. [CrossRef]
34. Puglisi, G.E.; Warzybok, A.; Hochmuth, S.; Visentin, C.; Astolfi, A.; Prodi, N.; Kollmeier, B. An Italian matrix sentence test for the evaluation of speech intelligibility in noise. *Int. J. Audiol.* **2015**, *54* (Suppl. S2), 44–50. [CrossRef]
35. Portelli, D.; Ciodaro, F.; Loteta, S.; Alberti, G.; Bruno, R. Audiological assessment with Matrix sentence test of percutaneous vs transcutaneous bone-anchored hearing aids: A pilot study. *Eur. Arch. Otorhinolaryngol.* **2023**, *Epub ahead of print*. [CrossRef]
36. Gazia, F.; Portelli, D.; Lo Vano, M.; Ciodaro, F.; Galletti, B.; Bruno, R.; Freni, F.; Alberti, G.; Galletti, F. Extended wear hearing aids: A comparative, pilot study. *Eur. Arch. Otorhinolaryngol.* **2022**, *279*, 5415–5422. [CrossRef]
37. Dobie, R.A. Prevention of Noise-Induced Hearing Loss. *Arch. Otolaryngol. Head Neck Surg.* **1995**, *121*, 385–391. [CrossRef]
38. Kwak, C.; Han, W. The Effectiveness of Hearing Protection Devices: A Systematic Review and Meta-Analysis. *Int. J. Environ. Res. Public Health* **2021**, *18*, 11693. [CrossRef]
39. Fu, V.X.; Oomens, P.; Merkus, N.; Jeekel, J. The Perception and Attitude Toward Noise and Music in the Operating Room: A Systematic Review. *J. Surg. Res.* **2021**, *263*, 193–206. [CrossRef]
40. Dholakia, S.; Jeans, J.P.; Khalid, U.; Dholakia, S.; D'Souza, C.; Nemeth, K. The association of noise and surgical-site infection in day-case hernia repairs. *Surgery* **2015**, *157*, 1153–1156. [CrossRef] [PubMed]
41. Kurmann, A.; Peter, M.; Tschan, F.; Mühlemann, K.; Candinas, D.; Beldi, G. Adverse effect of noise in the operating theatre on surgical-site infection. *Br. J. Surg.* **2011**, *98*, 1021–1025. [CrossRef] [PubMed]
42. Engelmann, C.R.; Neis, J.P.; Kirschbaum, C.; Grote, G.; Ure, B.M. A noise-reduction program in a pediatric operation theatre is associated with surgeon's benefits and a reduced rate of complications: A prospective controlled clinical trial. *Ann. Surg.* **2014**, *259*, 1025–1033. [CrossRef] [PubMed]
43. Jaszczak, A.; Pochodyła, E.; Kristianova, K.; Małkowska, N.; Kazak, J.K. Redefinition of Park Design Criteria as a Result of Analysis of Well-Being and Soundscape: The Case Study of the Kortowo Park (Poland). *Int. J. Environ. Res. Public Health* **2021**, *18*, 2972. [CrossRef]
44. Kohrman, D.; Wan, G.; Cassinotti, L.; Corfas, G. Hidden Hearing Loss: A Disorder with Multiple Etiologies and Mechanisms. *Cold Spring Harb. Perspect. Med.* **2020**, *10*, a035493. [CrossRef]

Disclaimer/Publisher's Note: The statements, opinions and data contained in all publications are solely those of the individual author(s) and contributor(s) and not of MDPI and/or the editor(s). MDPI and/or the editor(s) disclaim responsibility for any injury to people or property resulting from any ideas, methods, instructions or products referred to in the content.

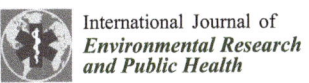

Article

Siblings' Risk of Adenoid Hypertrophy: A Cohort Study in Children

Aleksander Zwierz [1,*], Krzysztof Domagalski [2], Krystyna Masna [1] and Paweł Burduk [1]

1. Department of Otolaryngology, Phoniatrics and Audiology, Faculty of Health Sciences, Ludwik Rydygier Collegium Medicum, Nicolaus Copernicus University, 85-168 Bydgoszcz, Poland
2. Department of Immunology, Faculty of Biological and Veterinary Sciences, Nicolaus Copernicus University, 87-100 Torun, Poland
* Correspondence: aleksanderzwierz@gmail.com

Abstract: Background: The aim of this study was to compare adenoid size in preschool-age siblings using flexible nasopharyngoscopy examination (FNE) when they reach the same age. The occurrence of adenoid symptoms in these patients was also analyzed. This study was conducted to analyze the adenoid size in siblings when they reach the same age and substantiate a correlation between adenoid hypertrophy (AH) and adenoid symptoms. Methods: We analyzed and reported on the symptoms, ENT examination results, and FNE of 49 pairs of siblings who were examined at the same age. Results: There was a strong association in adenoid size between siblings when they are at a similar age (r = 0.673, $p < 0.001$). Second-born children whose older sibling had III° AH (A/C ratio > 65%) had a risk of III° AH 26 times greater than patients whose older sibling did not have III° AH (OR = 26.30, 95% CI = 2.82–245.54). Over 90% of snoring children whose siblings had confirmed III° AH would develop III° AH by the time they reach the same age. Second-born children in whom snoring occurs and whose older siblings have a III° AH have about a 46 times higher risk of III° AH compared to patients who did not meet these two conditions ($p < 0.001$, OR = 46.67, 95% CI = 8.37–260.30). Conclusions: A significant familial correlation between adenoid size in siblings when they reach the same age was shown. If the older sibling has a confirmed overgrown adenoid (III° AH) and their younger sibling presents adenoid symptoms, particularly snoring, it is highly probable that they will also have an overgrown adenoid.

Keywords: adenoid hypertrophy; AH; siblings; flexible nasopharyngoscopy; adenoid symptoms

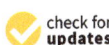

Citation: Zwierz, A.; Domagalski, K.; Masna, K.; Burduk, P. Siblings' Risk of Adenoid Hypertrophy: A Cohort Study in Children. *Int. J. Environ. Res. Public Health* **2023**, *20*, 2910. https://doi.org/10.3390/ijerph20042910

Academic Editors: Francesco Gazia, Bruno Galletti, Gay-Escoda Cosme, Francesco Ciodaro and Rocco Bruno

Received: 22 December 2022
Revised: 2 February 2023
Accepted: 7 February 2023
Published: 7 February 2023

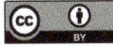

Copyright: © 2023 by the authors. Licensee MDPI, Basel, Switzerland. This article is an open access article distributed under the terms and conditions of the Creative Commons Attribution (CC BY) license (https:// creativecommons.org/licenses/by/ 4.0/).

1. Introduction

Adenoid hypertrophy (AH) is one of the most common diseases among preschool children, usually associated with adenoid symptoms, such as mouth breathing, persistent rhinitis, snoring, and a nasal voice [1]. If the disease presents in an older child of a family, parents will often suspect that the same symptoms described above will resurface later in a younger sibling in the family. A common question is whether this problem is familial, especially if the parents also underwent or were considered as a child for adenoidectomy. In 1980, Katznelson and Gross first confirmed a significantly higher incidence of prior tonsillectomy and adenoidectomy performed on an analyzed group of siblings and parents than controls [2]. However, all later performed analyses and surgical procedures were based on presented adenoid symptoms, not on a true measurement of adenoid size. Thus, it is difficult to compare parents and their children, because diagnostic techniques have changed and improved over the years. Nowadays, flexible nasopharyngoscopy examination (FNE) seems the gold standard, not only for assessing adenoid size but also for checking the mucus coverage of the adenoid [3].

It is commonly believed that the adenoid undergoes hypertrophy during childhood, and eventually, involution in adulthood [4]. Over the years, several longitudinal studies, Handelman and Osborne (1976), Ishida et al. (2018), and Yamada et al. (2021), have assessed the size of the adenoid using lateral cephalometric radiography [5–7]. Yamada showed that an overgrowth of adenoids occurred in preschool children, but there were no significant changes in the adenoid size from 8–12 years of age [7]. A previous study based on flexible endoscopic examinations revealed that adenoid involution proceeds rather slowly; only 7.9% of preschool children (aged 3–7 years) underwent a change in the adenoid size by >15% on the adenoid to choana (A/C) ratio over one year of observation, 21.6% over a period of 2 years, and 45% over a period of 3 years [8]. The growth and development patterns of the nasopharyngeal lymphoid tissues vary for each individual; accordingly, we believe that in studies comparing the adenoid size in a pair of siblings, the permissible age difference should not exceed 12 months.

This study aimed to compare the adenoid size of siblings who were raised in the same household. In most cases, the pairs of children studied were raised with exposure to the same environmental factors, such as cigarette smoke, pollution, and mold allergens, which are considered risk factors for the development of AH [9,10]. Tobacco smoke exposure has been particularly reported as a risk factor for AH [10]; however, nowadays, numerous preventive campaigns have been conducted in our country, and parents are abundantly aware of the risks associated with cigarette smoke exposure in children. Therefore, there is a common practice of avoiding smoking in rooms where children reside. Nevertheless, parents who violate this rule will usually not admit it. Furthermore, the city and rural living conditions may vary in terms of air pollution and allergen exposure, so we analyzed the influence of area of residence on AH. Notably, the duration of breastfeeding is a potential factor distinguishing between babies living in one environment, and breastfeeding has been indicated as a risk factor for snoring and obstructive sleep apnea syndrome (OSAS) [11–13]. Xu et al. stated this correlation and highlighted the need for further investigations to confirm the relationship between breastfeeding and OSAS and the mechanisms underlying it [11]. Chng et al. suggest that breastfeeding independently increases the risk of snoring and possible obstructive sleep apnea syndrome [12]. In another study, Montgomery-Downs et al. indicated that OSAS severity is reduced in association with breastfeeding, but it should not be interpreted to suggest that breastfeeding entirely prevents the development of sleep disorder breathing [13]. Presumably, AH may be operational in this mechanism; however, to the best of our knowledge, no study has confirmed a relationship between breastfeeding and AH. Moreover, no genetic factors associated with AH have been discovered so far to demonstrate a similarity in the adenoid size of siblings and justify further research.

FNE is a common procedure to evaluate adenoid size, and this study used FNE to compare adenoid sizes in siblings when they reach the same age. This study was conducted to analyze the adenoid size in siblings when they reach the same age and substantiate a correlation between AH and adenoid symptoms.

2. Materials and Methods

2.1. Study Population

We retrospectively analyzed a group of 1247 preschool children (3–7 year of age) who visited a medical outpatient ear, nose, and throat (ENT) clinic with symptoms suggestive of chronic AH between 2016 and 2021. We searched the medical history of all preschool children admitted to the ENT outpatient clinic. Then, 82 pairs of siblings were selected. We included in the study each pair of children if they were examined in the ENT outpatient clinic at around the same age, where the permissible age difference should not exceed 12 months. We then called their caretakers to confirm if the siblings had the same parents. Exclusion criteria from the study were: children brought up in a common household who have the same last name but different parents, craniofacial anomalies, such as cleft lip/cleft palate; genetic diseases (Down Syndrome); septal nasal deviation; nasal polyp or inferior turbinate hypertrophy; active upper respiratory infection within 2 weeks of enrolling in the study; or previously performed adenoidectomy. In the end, 49 pairs of siblings qualified for participation in the study.

The initial assessment of each patient after study enrollment included a parental questionnaire concerning recurrent upper respiratory infections, defined as a frequent runny nose, pharyngitis, or a cough [14]. We also analyzed the symptoms of rhinitis—at least two nasal symptoms: rhinorrhea, blockage, sneezing, or itching and snoring—defined as persistent, occasional, or non-existent [15]. All children performed an ENT physical examination, flexible fiberoptic rhinoscopy, and tympanometry.

Additionally, we analyzed whether residing in the city or rural regions affects the adenoid size. We divided the children into two groups: those living in the city (population: 170,000–340,000 citizens), and those living in the countryside.

Seasons may influence adenoid mucus coverage and tympanometry type [3]. To avoid any seasonal influence on the obtained results and compare better the sibling population from this study, we divided the year into two main seasons, winter and summer, and we considered the cut-off temperature to be 10 °C and also analyzed seasons of performed examination.

2.2. Endoscopy

Each child underwent flexible endoscopic examinations using common nasal meatus, performed by one pediatric otorhinolaryngologist (A.Z.) using the Karl Storz Tele Pack endoscopic system, which was equipped with a flexible nasopharyngoscope (2.8-mm outer diameter and 300-mm length). The percentages of obturation (adenoid-to-choanae ratio in percentage-A/C ratio) of the choanae and mucus coverage of the adenoids were analyzed based on videoendoscopy with the freeze-frame option. Choanal obstructions were assessed with an accuracy of up to 5%. For a better statistical assessment, patients were divided into groups for which we used the 3-degree Bolesławska scale, particularly the part concerning adenoid size in relation to the nasopharynx [16]. All recorded videos of the nasopharynx were coded and blindly analyzed. The percentage of choanal obstruction by the adenoid was measured and compared between siblings. Adenoid size and mucus coverage recorded on the endoscopic system were compared by a second doctor (K.M.). If there was a discrepancy in the assessment, the score was reassessed by a third ENT doctor (P.B.).

The difference in adenoid size between each sibling pair was considered a percentage difference in the amount of nasopharyngeal obstruction by the adenoid. In addition, we used the previous proposed scale to assess the mucus coverage of the adenoid, called the Mucus of Adenoid Scale by Nasopharyngoscopy Assessment (MASNA), which describes the amount of mucus covering the adenoid on a four-point scale (0, no mucus; 1, residue of clear watery mucus; 2, some amount of dense mucus; 3, copious thick dense mucus) [3].

2.3. Tympanometry

An otoscopic examination was performed, and if needed, the external auditory canal was cleaned. In addition, tympanometry was performed using the GSI 39 Auto Tymp™ by Grason-Stadler. The middle ear effusion in each ear was analyzed by tympanometry measurement, and tympanogram graphs were generated. The results were classified using the classification system for tympanograms developed by Liden and Jerger [17,18]. The sequence of saved tympanograms for each patient ear was right, left. We posit that type-B tympanograms produced the worst result, type-C, significant negative pressure in the middle ear, was worse, and type-A, normal middle ear status, was good. For a further statistical analysis, we divided the children into three groups, considering the worse tympanogram result for each child: Group A children with type-A tympanogram in both ears (AA), group C children with tympanogram C (CC, AC, and CA), and group B children with tympanogram B (BB, BC, CB, AB, and BA).

2.4. Ethics

Ethical approval for this study was obtained by the ethics committee of Nicolaus Copernicus University (KB 559/2021).

2.5. Statistical Analysis

We used descriptive statistics to summarize and describe the variables for the study group. We summarized quantitative variables, such as age and adenoid size, based on their means ± standard deviations (SDs). For the categorical variables, we used frequency counts and percentages. To determine differences between variables, statistical significance was estimated using the Chi-square method or Fisher's exact test for categorical variables and the Student's t-test or ANOVA for quantitative variables. Associations between variables were analyzed using Pearson's correlation.

Variables significantly related to adenoid size in a univariate analysis were included in the linear and logistic regression analyses. The linear regression analysis assessed variables of significance for the prediction of adenoid size (A/C ratio, %) volatility in the whole study group. In our linear regression analysis, variables such as recurrent upper respiratory tract infections, rhinitis, snoring, adenoid mucus coverage, and type of tympanogram were assigned appropriate values (for recurrent upper respiratory tract infections (rURTI), rhinitis, snoring: 0, symptom not present; 1, symptom present; for adenoid mucus coverage: from 0 to 4 according MASNA scale; for tympanogram type: 0–A, 1–C, 2–B).

To check for any differences between the pairs of analyzed siblings, the children were divided into two groups: the first including the first examined child from the pair, usually the older of the siblings, and the second including the second examined child, usually the younger. If large families were analyzed, only one pair of siblings from a given family was preferred. We selected the sibling pair with the smallest age difference at the time of examinations.

To analyze the associations between a significant increase in adenoid size (AH) in the second-born child and clinical factors, such as recurrent upper respiratory tract infections, rhinitis, snoring, adenoid mucus coverage, and tympanogram type as categorical variables, a logistic regression analysis was performed. III° AH was defined as an A/C ratio of >65%, based on the Bolesławska scale, where 65% is the cut-off point between II° and III° AH. To predict an A/C ratio of >65% in second-born children, we conducted two separate assessments of: (1) second-born factors and (2) second-born factors and first-born adenoid size. Odds ratios (ORs) and 95% confidence intervals (95% CIs) were also calculated for the considered clinical variables in the regression models.

For all these tests, two-tailed p-values were used, and differences at the level of $p < 0.05$ were considered significant. All statistical analyses were performed using the SPSS (Statistical Package for the Social Sciences version 26, Armonk, NY, USA) software.

3. Results

The mean age of the first examined child group was 5.0 years (SD = 2.2), and that of the second examined child group was 5.1 (SD = 2.2). The mean adenoid size as an A/C ratio for the first sample was 63%, and it was 59% for the second. In total, 71.4% of parents reported rURTI in the first group of siblings and 51% in the second. Rhinitis was present in 77.6% of children from the first group and in 65.3% from the second group. Persistent and occasional snoring were present in, respectively, 36.7% and 28.6% of children from the first group and 34.7% and 26.5% from the second group. Mucous coverage of the adenoid according to MASNA scale grades 0 to 3 was, respectively, 30.6%, 44.9%, 18.4%, and 6.1% in the first group and 28.6%, 38.8%, 24.5%, and 8.2% in the second group. Analyzing the tympanometry results, we found 53.1% type-A tympanograms, 20.4% type-C tympanograms, and 26.5% type-B tympanograms in the first group and 67.3% type-A tympanograms, 12.2% type-C tympanograms, and 20.4% type-B tympanograms in the second group. Comparing examinations in thermal seasons, 42.9% of children were examined in the summer and 57.1% in the winter in the first group and 55.1% in the summer and 44.9% in the winter in the second group. No differences between groups were found in terms of the analyzed data, except rURTI. All presented data are included in Table 1.

Table 1. Demographic and clinical characteristics of study population according to birth order of siblings.

Characteristic		First-Born Children	Second-Born Children	p Value
n		49	49	
Age (years)	Mean ± SD	5.0 ± 2.2	5.1 ± 2.2	0.110
	Median (Q25–Q75)	4.3 (3.7–5.6)	4.6 (3.6–5.7)	
Sex	Female	23 (46.9%)	15 (30.6%)	0.134
	Male	26 (53.1%)	34 (69.4%)	
rURTI *	No	14 (28.6%)	24 (49.0%)	0.021
	Yes	35 (71.4%)	25 (51.0%)	
Rhinitis	No	11 (22.4%)	17 (34.7%)	0.210
	Yes	38 (77.6%)	32 (65.3%)	
Snoring	No	17 (34.7%)	13 (26.5%)	0.630
	Occasionally	14 (28.6%)	19 (38.8%)	
	Persistent	18 (36.7%)	17 (34.7%)	
Adenoid size (A/C ratio and (Bolesławska scale, %)	Mean ± SD	63.0 ± 17	59.0 ± 20	0.163
	Median (Q25–Q75)	60.0 (50.0–75.0)	60.0 (50.0–75.0)	
	<35 (B I)	2 (4.1%)	6 (12.2%)	
	35–65 (B II)	27 (55.1%)	25 (51.0%)	0.396
	>65 (B III)	20 (40.8%)	18 (36.7%)	
Adenoid mucus coverage (MASNA scale)	0	15 (30.6%)	14 (28.6%)	
	1	22 (44.9%)	19 (38.8%)	0.387
	2	9 (18.4%)	12 (24.5%)	
	3	3 (6.1%)	4 (8.2%)	
Tympanogram	AA	26 (53.1%)	33 (67.3%)	
	AB/BA	2 (4.1%)	0 (0.0%)	
	AC/CA	5 (10.2%)	4 (8.2%)	-
	BB	10 (20.4%)	7 (14.3%)	
	CB/BC	1 (2.0%)	3 (6.2%)	
	CC	5 (10.2%)	2 (4.1%)	
	A	26 (53.1%)	33 (67.3%)	
	B	13 (26.5%)	10 (20.4%)	0.340
	C	10 (20.4%)	6 (12.2%)	
Thermal season	Summer	21 (42.9%)	27 (55.1%)	0.263
	Winter	28 (57.1%)	22 (44.9%)	

* rURTI—recurrent upper respiratory tract infections.

An association between adenoid size in siblings was determined by Pearson's correlation analysis. The correlation coefficient between adenoid size on the A/C ratio between the first- and the second-born siblings showed a strong positive association (r = 0.673, p < 0.001 (Figure 1).

In the next analysis step, the relationships between demographic or clinical factors and adenoid size were analyzed for the entire group of children (Table 2). Statistically significant differences in A/C ratios were obtained for rURTI (p < 0.001), rhinitis (p < 0.001), snoring (p < 0.001), tympanometry type (p < 0.001), and adenoid mucus coverage (p = 0.002). Patients with rURTI and rhinitis, snoring, impaired tympanogram, or high adenoid mucus coverage according to the MASNA scale had an increased A/C ratio. There were no associations between adenoid size and sex and seasonality. Moreover, we analyzed adenoid size change according to age for the whole patient sample (Figure 2). A linear correlation analysis showed no significant correlation between age and adenoid size (r = −0.125, p = 0.219). We also analyzed the living conditions (in the city or countryside) as an environmental factor influencing the adenoid size. No significant correlation between adenoid size in children living in city and countryside was found.

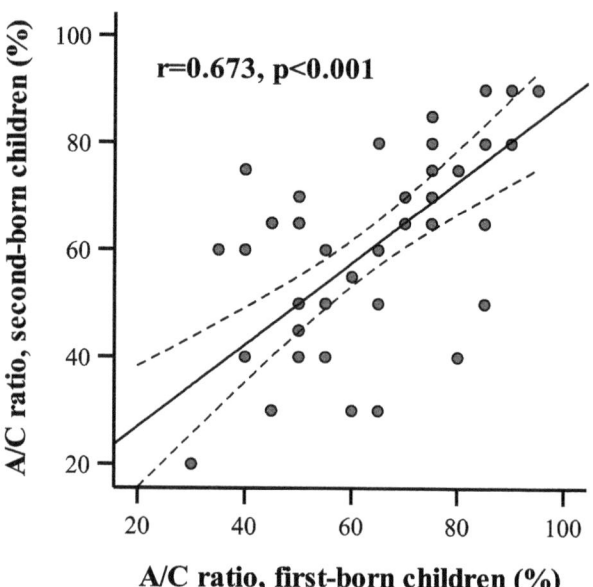

Figure 1. A/C ratio correlation between the first- and second-born children in the family.

Table 2. Relationships between demographic or clinical factors and adenoid size in children with symptoms suggestive of chronic AH.

Characteristic (n = 98)		Adenoid Size (A/C Ratio), % Mean ± SD	p Value
Sex	Female	64.1 ± 20.5	0.195
	Male	59.1 ± 17.1	
rURTI	No	50.0 ± 15.9	<0.001
	Yes	68.0 ± 16.7	
Rhinitis	No	51.6 ± 15.6	0.001
	Yes	64.8 ± 18.3	
Snoring	No	50.5 ± 19.3	<0.001
	Occasionally	60.0 ± 15.4	
	Persistent	71.0 ± 15.4	
	No	50.5 ± 19.3	<0.001
	Yes	65.7 ± 16.3	
Adenoid mucus coverage (MASNA scale)	0	52.8 ± 18.2	0.002
	1	60.0 ± 18.1	
	2	70.2 ± 15.8	
	3	73.6 ± 13.5	
Tympanogram	A	54.5 ± 17.8	<0.001
	B	74.6 ± 15.2	
	C	65.6 ± 13.5	
	A	54.5 ± 17.8	<0.001
	Non-A	70.9 ± 15.0	
Thermal season	Summer	58.2 ± 19.8	0.145
	Winter	63.7 ± 17.0	
Place of residence	countryside	59.8 ± 19.9	0.901
	city	60.3 ± 19.4	

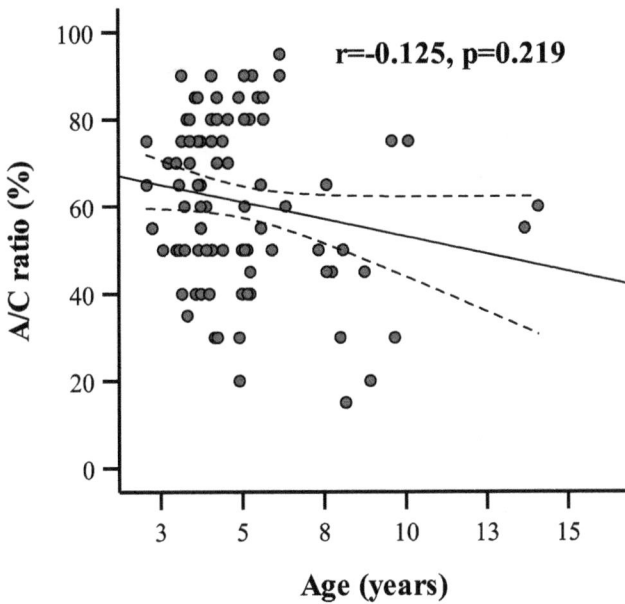

Figure 2. Correlation between A/C ratio and age of study population ($n = 98$).

Variables significantly related to adenoid size in the univariate analysis were included in the linear and logistic regression analyses to identify independent prognostic factors useful in assessing adenoid size. Linear regression analysis for predicting the adenoid size variance in the whole study group revealed that rURTI, snoring, adenoid mucus coverage, and tympanogram type impact the assessment of adenoid size, but not rhinitis (Table 3). Interestingly, the most important aspect is whether the patient is snoring ($\beta = 0.329$), followed by the tympanogram type ($\beta = 0.269$).

Table 3. Linear regression analysis for the prediction of adenoid size in children ($n = 98$).

Characteristic	p Value	B with 95% CI	Beta (β)
rURTI	0.015	9.04 (1.81–16.27)	0.24
Rhinitis	0.470	2.73 (−4.74–10.20)	0.07
Snoring	<0.001	7.47 (3.94–10.99)	0.33
Adenoid mucus coverage	0.019	3.98 (.67–7.30)	0.19
Tympanogram	0.001	6.25 (2.58–9.92)	0.27

The main analysis in this study focused on assessing the significance of clinical factors in the prognosis of III° AH in siblings. For this, logistic regression analyses for the detection of III° AH (A/C ratio > 65%) in second-born children were performed. Using second-born child factors, logistic regression analyses showed importance only for snoring ($p = 0.006$) and tympanogram type ($p = 0.029$; Table 4). Patients diagnosed with snoring have more than a 6-fold greater risk of III° AH (OR = 6.23, 95% CI = 1.7–22.70) compared to patients who do not snore. Likewise, the presence of an ear impairment demonstrated by type-B or -C tympanogram relates to an over 6-fold increase in the risk of III° AH (OR = 6.30, 95% CI = 1.20–32.99).

Table 4. Logistic regression analysis for the prediction of III° AH (A/C ratio > 65%) in second-born children ($n = 49$).

Characteristic	p Value	OR	95% CI
Second-born child factors			
rURTI, yes	0.736	1.37	0.22–8.43
Rhinitis, yes	0.897	1.14	0.15–8.57
Snoring, yes	0.006	6.23	1.7–22.70
Adenoid mucus coverage (MASNA scale), per category	0.14	1.96	0.80–4.79
Tympanogram, non-A	0.029	6.30	1.20–32.99
Second-born child factors and adenoid size of the first-born child			
rURTI, yes	0.543	0.48	0.04–5.15
Rhinitis, yes	0.575	2.05	0.17–25.08
Snoring, yes	0.015	8.43	1.51–46.95
Adenoid mucus coverage (MASNA scale), per category	0.335	1.68	0.59–4.81
Tympanogram, non-A	0.178	4.34	0.51–36.77
Adenoid size of the first-born child, A/C ratio > 65%	0.004	26.30	2.82–245.54

As shown, there was a strong association in adenoid size between siblings at a similar age. Therefore, we subsequently analyzed the importance of adenoid size in older siblings in relation to assessing adenoid size in younger siblings using logistic regression analysis. For this analysis, the adenoid size of the first-born child was categorized as the binary clinical variable (A/C ratio $\leq$ 65% vs. >65%). According to the assumed criterion, an A/C ratio of >65% was detected in 20 first-born children (40.8%). The logistic regression analysis showed that the assumed variable had the strongest significant effect on the prediction of III° AH ($p = 0.004$; Table 4). The obtained estimates indicate that second-born children whose older siblings had III° AH had more than a 26-fold greater risk of III° AH compared to patients whose older sibling did not have III° AH (OR = 26.30, 95% CI = 2.82–245.54). In addition to the adenoid size of the first-born child, from all the analyzed factors that affected the second-born child, only snoring was shown to be a predictive factor of III° AH in the younger sibling ($p = 0.015$, OR = 8.43, 95% CI = 1.51–46.95). The resulting data showed that knowledge of adenoid size in older siblings eliminates the importance of type of tympanogram in the younger child to estimate their risk of III° AH.

Finally, we assess the potential predictive value of snoring in the second-born child by relating it with an A/C ratio of >65% in the first-born child. Over 90% of snoring children whose sibling had confirmed III° AH would later develop III° AH (Table 5). In our series, second-born children in whom snoring occurs and whose older siblings have a known A/C ratio of >65% have about a 46-fold higher risk of III° AH (A/C > 65%) compared to patients who did not meet these two conditions ($p < 0.001$, OR = 46,67, 95% CI = 8.37–260.30) (Table 5).

Table 5. The relationship between snoring in the second-born child and an A/C ratio of >65% in the first-born child and an A/C ratio > 65% in the second-born children group with symptoms suggestive of chronic AH.

		Adenoid Size (A/C Ratio, %) of the Second-Born Child		p Value	OR (95% CI)
		$\leq$65	>65		
Snoring in the second-born child and A/C ratio > 65% in the first-born child	yes	28 (90.3%)	3 (16.7%)	<0.001	46.67 (8.37–260.30)
	no	3 (9.7%)	15 (83.3%)		

These results indicate that combining snoring in second-born children with adenoid size in first-born children in the same family clearly improves the prediction of III° AH in second-born patients.

4. Discussion

Our work shows a significant correlation between adenoid size in siblings if an FNE is performed at the same age. Katznelson and Gross observed a difference in the number of adenoidectomies between operated parents and siblings and the control group, which might suggest a familial susceptibility to AH [2]. On the other hand, the authors suggest that parents who were previously operated on or who have a child who was previously operated on might be more willing to allow the surgery to be performed on their second child. Still, our results confirmed the hypothesis of familial susceptibility to hypertrophy based on endoscopically assessed adenoid size. However, Bani-Ata et al. indicated a low significance of tonsillectomy in parental and sibling histories [19], but the size of palatine tonsils is not the main indication for tonsillectomy; therefore, it is difficult to compare a family predisposition to adenoidectomy with tonsillectomy. However, recurrent or chronic inflammation susceptibility of the adenoids or palatine tonsil tissue may lead to chronic activation of the cell-mediated and humoral immune response, which may play a role in hypertrophy [20]. This susceptibility to infection may be caused by genetic dispositions. The role of different variations in inflammatory genetic factors, such as polymorphisms of mannose binding lectin (MBL), toll-like receptors (TLRs), secretoglobulins (SCGBs), or IL-10, were analyzed [20–23]. Grasso et al. found that the MBL2 00 genotype is a prognostic marker of AH in children [21]. Meanwhile, Babademez et al. stated that *TLR4* polymorphisms were associated with an increased risk of AH, but they did not find the same association when they analyzed *TLR2* polymorphisms [20]. In addition, in the work of Özdaş et al., the presence of single nucleotide polymorphisms (SNPs) of secretoglobulins were associated with an increased risk of AH [22]. Another study demonstrated the role of the *IL-10* genotype GG in resistance to hypertrophy [23]. All these data support the hypothesis that the inheritance of AH is likely polygenic, involving aspects of physiology determined by multiple genes. Moreover, other non-genetic (environmental) factors, such as cytomegalovirus, human herpesvirus type 6, and infections, may play a role in AH [23]. These factors may co-occur in siblings from the same family who are in constant contact with each other. A study performed by Trask et al. shows that both allergic and non-allergic sibling groups showed a larger mean adenoid size on radiographs than controls [24].

Our study offers practical knowledge for pediatricians. Snoring children have a 6-fold greater risk of AH (III° in Bolesławska scale, A/C ratio > 65%) compared to patients who do not snore. In addition, children with an abnormal (not type-A) tympanogram and indirect effusion in the middle ear indicated a six-times greater chance of III° AH compared to children with a type-A tympanogram. The obtained results indicate that second-born children whose older sibling had III° AH have more than a 26-fold greater risk of III° AH compared to patients whose older siblings do not have AH. Second-born children will have a 46-fold increased chance of developing III° AH if they snore and if their older sibling has previously confirmed III° AH.

AH is the one of the main etiological factors for pediatric sleep disordered breathing (SDB). Lundkvist et al. analyzed parents affected by obstructive sleep apnea (OSAS) and their children, and they concluded that children whose parents were affected by OSAS had a substantially higher risk of hospitalization for SDB [25]. These symptoms were associated with pediatric OSAS or either adenoid or palatine tonsillar hypertrophy. Carmelli et al. analyzed genetic factors in self-reported snoring and excessive daytime sleepiness in twins, arguing that the inheritance of sleep apnea symptoms may be polygenic, but it can also be modulated by the environmental factors in which the twins grow up [26]. The issue of OSAS and hypertrophy of the adenoid and palatine tonsils in siblings was also analyzed by Friberg [27], who showed a significant risk of OSAS in children whose sibling has an OSAS diagnosis, significantly higher than in children with adenoid and palatine tonsils hypertrophy. This study, database research that analyzed AH, was based on a medical diagnosis described in the patient medical history by the ICD-10 code.

In addition, we showed in the whole analyzed group of children a correlation between adenoid size and such adenoid symptoms and related illnesses as rURTI, rhinitis, snoring, poor mucus coverage, and poor tympanometry type. This confirms the role of III° AH in the mentioned factors also described by other authors [1,28–31].

In our study, we showed a close relationship between AH in children and snoring. We stated that involution of the adenoid in children who snore and who have AH decreases slowly and linearly (Figure 2). The shape of the curve on the graph is similar to that presented by Papaioannou et al. [32]. They analyzed adenoid size in an MRI study in children of different ages and concluded that in children who do not snore, adenoid size increases to 7–8 years of age and then it slowly decreases (parabolic curve), and in the group of children who snore (more than 1 night per week), the reduction in adenoid size occurred slowly until 18 years (linear curve).

In summary, this study shows a great familial correlation between adenoid size in siblings based on real adenoid sizes measured by FNE. Other similar studies were based on a history of performed surgery and reported symptoms or ICD-10 code. Due to a lack of a historical possibility to analyze adenoid size via an endoscopic examination in parents because this technology was unavailable when parents were at their children's age, only endoscopic images of siblings' adenoids were comparable.

A limitation in this study was the difficulty of selection of siblings who were examined at the same age, because some parents whose older child was diagnosed with AH or who had presented adenoid symptoms and related illness decided to diagnose their younger child earlier and, based on their own experience earlier, opted for surgery. The influence on sample size is related to the fact that this group was examined by one children's ENT specialist (A.Z.) in the same ENT outpatient clinic. Further, the repeatability of the tests performed is affected by the use of the same doctor using the same flexible endoscopic system.

5. Conclusions

We showed a significant familial correlation between adenoid size in siblings when they reach the same age. The obtained result indicates the environmental and genetic mechanisms of AH, but due to the polygenicity of the issue, more research is necessary.

Our results also suggest that experiences and observations related to the medical history and examination of the older child can be helpful in making a timely diagnosis of the younger child. It is especially important for pediatricians to consider that when an older sibling has a confirmed overgrown adenoid (III° AH) and their younger sibling presents adenoid symptoms, particularly snoring, it is highly probable that they will also have an overgrown adenoid (46 times greater risk).

Author Contributions: Conceptualization, A.Z. and K.D.; methodology, A.Z. and K.D.; software, K.D.; validation, A.Z. and K.D.; formal analysis, A.Z. and K.D.; investigation, A.Z. and K.M.; resources, A.Z.; data curation, A.Z. and K.M.; writing—original draft preparation, A.Z. and K.D.; writing—review and editing, A.Z.; visualization, A.Z.; supervision, P.B.; project administration, A.Z.; All authors have read and agreed to the published version of the manuscript.

Funding: This research received no external funding.

Institutional Review Board Statement: Ethical approval for this study was obtained from the ethics committee of Nicolaus Copernicus University (KB 136/2022). Date of approval 15.02.2022.

Informed Consent Statement: Informed consent was obtained from all subjects involved in the study.

Data Availability Statement: Additional data supporting reported results may be available for request.

Conflicts of Interest: The authors declare no conflict of interest.

References

1. Marseglia, G.; Caimmi, D.; Pagella, F.; Matti, E.; Labò, E.; Licari, A.; Salpietro, A.; Pelizzo, G.; Castellazzi, A. Adenoids during childhood: The facts. *Int. J. Immunopathol. Pharmacol.* **2011**, *24* (Suppl. 4), 1–5. [CrossRef] [PubMed]
2. Katznelson, D.; Gross, S. Familial clustering of tonsillectomies and adenoidectomies. *Clin. Pediatr.* **1980**, *19*, 276–283. [CrossRef] [PubMed]
3. Masna, K.; Zwierz, A.; Domagalski, K.; Burduk, P. The impact of the thermal seasons on adenoid size, its mucus coverage and otitis media with effusion: A cohort study. *J. Clin. Med.* **2021**, *10*, 5603. [CrossRef] [PubMed]
4. Harris, J.A.; Jackson, C.M.; Paterson, D.G.; Scammon, S.E. *The Measurement of the Body in Childhood in the Measurement of Man*; University of Minnesota Press: Minneapolis, MN, USA, 1930.
5. Ishida, T.; Manabe, A.; Yang, S.S.; Yoon, H.S.; Kanda, E.; Ono, T. Patterns of adenoid and tonsil growth in Japanese children and adolescents: A longitudinal study. *Sci. Rep.* **2018**, *8*, 17088. [CrossRef] [PubMed]
6. Handelman, C.S.; Osborne, G. Growth of the nasopharynx and adenoid development from one to eighteen years. *Angle Orthod.* **1976**, *46*, 243–259.
7. Yamada, H.; Sawada, M.; Higashino, M.; Abe, S.; El-Bialy, T.; Tanaka, E. Longitudinal Morphological Changes in the Adenoids and Tonsils in Japanese School Children. *J. Clin. Med.* **2021**, *10*, 4956. [CrossRef]
8. Zwierz, A.; Domagalski, K.; Masna, K.; Burduk, P. Effectiveness of Evaluation of Adenoid Hypertrophy in Children by Flexible Nasopharyngoscopy Examination (FNE), Proposed Schema of Frequency of Examination: Cohort Study. *Diagnostics* **2022**, *12*, 1734. [CrossRef]
9. Huang, S.W.; Giannoni, C. The risk of adenoid hypertrophy in children with allergic rhinitis. *Ann. Allergy Asthma Immunol.* **2001**, *87*, 350–355. [CrossRef]
10. Evcimik, M.F.; Dogru, M.; Cirik, A.A.; Nepesov, M.I. Adenoid hypertrophy in children with allergic disease and influential factors. *Int. J. Pediatr. Otorhinolaryngol.* **2015**, *79*, 694–697. [CrossRef]
11. Xu, Z.; Wu, Y.; Tai, J.; Feng, G.; Ge, W.; Zheng, L.; Zhou, Z.; Ni, X. Risk factors of obstructive sleep apnea syndrome in children. *J. Otolaryngol. Head Neck Surg.* **2020**, *49*, 11. [CrossRef]
12. Chng, S.Y.; Goh, D.Y.; Wang, X.S.; Tan, T.N.; Ong, N.B. Snoring and atopic disease: A strong association. *Pediatr. Pulmonol.* **2004**, *38*, 210–216. [CrossRef] [PubMed]
13. Montgomery-Downs, H.E.; Crabtree, V.M.; Sans Capdevila, O.; Gozal, D. Infant-feeding methods and childhood sleep-disordered breathing. *Pediatrics* **2007**, *120*, 1030–1035. [CrossRef] [PubMed]
14. Bonfim, C.M.; Nogueira, M.L.; Simas, P.V.M.; Gardinassi, L.G.A.; Durigon, E.L.; Rahal, P.; Souza, F.P. Frequent respiratory pathogens of respiratory tract infections in children attending daycare centers. *J. Pediatr. (Rio J.)* **2011**, *87*, 439–444. (In English, Portuguese) [CrossRef] [PubMed]
15. Roberts, G.; Xatzipsalti, M.; Borrego, L.M.; Custovic, A.; Halken, S.; Hellings, P.; Papadopoulos, N.; Rotiroti, G.; Scadding, G.; Timmermans, F.; et al. Paediatric rhinitis: Position paper of the European Academy of Allergy and Clinical Immunology. *Allergy* **2013**, *68*, 1102–1116. [CrossRef]
16. Boleslavská, J.; Koprivová, H.; Komínek, P. Is it important to evaluate the size of adenoid vegetations? *Otorinolaryngol. Foniatr.* **2006**, *55*, 133–138. (In Czech)
17. Lidén, G. The scope and application of current audiometric tests. *J. Laryngol. Otol.* **1969**, *83*, 507–520. [CrossRef]
18. Jerger, J. Clinical experience with impedance audiometry. *Arch. Otolaryngol.* **1970**, *92*, 311–324. [CrossRef]
19. Bani-Ata, M.; Aleshawi, A.; Alali, M.; Kanaan, Y.; Al-Momani, W.; Kanaan, N.; Abdalla, K.; Alhowary, A. familial and environmental risk predisposition in tonsillectomy: A case-control study. *Risk Manag. Healthc. Policy* **2020**, *13*, 847–853. [CrossRef]
20. Babademez, M.A.; Özdaş, T.; Özdaş, S. The common genetic variants of toll-like receptor and susceptibility to adenoid hypertrophy: A hospital-based cohort study. *Turk. J. Med. Sci.* **2016**, *46*, 1449–1458. [CrossRef]
21. Grasso, D.L.; Guerci, V.I.; Zocconi, E.; Milanese, M.; Segat, L.; Crovella, S. MBL2 genetic polymorphisms in Italian children with adenotonsillar hypertrophy. *Int. J. Pediatr. Otorhinolaryngol.* **2007**, *71*, 1013–1016. [CrossRef] [PubMed]
22. Özdaş, T.; Özdaş, S.; Babademez, M.A.; Muz, S.E.; Atilla, M.H.; Baştimur, S.; Izbirak, G.; Kurt, K.; Öz, I. Significant association between SCGB1D4 gene polymorphisms and susceptibility to adenoid hypertrophy in a pediatric population. *Turk. J. Med. Sci.* **2017**, *47*, 201–210. [CrossRef]
23. Lomaeva, I.; Aghajanyan, A.; Dzhaparidze, L.; Gigani, O.B.; Tskhovrebova, L.V.; Gigani, O.O.; Popadyuk, V.I. Adenoid hypertrophy risk in children carriers of G-1082A polymorphism of IL-10 infected with human herpes virus (HHV6, EBV, CMV). *Life* **2022**, *12*, 266. [CrossRef] [PubMed]
24. Trask, G.M.; Shapiro, G.G.; Shapiro, P.A. The effects of perennial allergic rhinitis on dental and skeletal development: A comparison of sibling pairs. *Am. J. Orthod. Dentofac. Orthop.* **1987**, *92*, 286–293. [CrossRef] [PubMed]
25. Lundkvist, K.; Sundquist, K.; Li, X.; Friberg, D. Familial risk of sleep-disordered breathing. *Sleep Med.* **2012**, *13*, 668–673. [CrossRef] [PubMed]
26. Carmelli, D.; Bliwise, D.L.; Swan, G.E.; Reed, T. Genetic factors in self-reported snoring and excessive daytime sleepiness: A twin study. *Am. J. Respir. Crit. Care Med.* **2001**, *164*, 949–952. [CrossRef] [PubMed]
27. Friberg, D.; Sundquist, J.; Li, X.; Hemminki, K.; Sundquist, K. Sibling risk of pediatric obstructive sleep apnea syndrome and adenotonsillar hypertrophy. *Sleep* **2009**, *32*, 1077–1083. [CrossRef]

28. Berçin, A.S.; Ural, A.; Kutluhan, A.; Yurttaş, V. Relationship between sinusitis and adenoid size in pediatric age group. *Ann. Otol. Rhinol. Laryngol.* **2007**, *116*, 550–553. [CrossRef]
29. Dixit, Y.; Tripathi, P.S. Community level evaluation of adenoid hypertrophy on the basis of symptom scoring and its X-ray correlation. *J. Fam. Med. Prim. Care* **2016**, *5*, 789–791.
30. Gulotta, G.; Iannella, G.; Vicini, C.; Polimeni, A.; Greco, A.; De Vincentiis, M.; Visconti, I.C.; Meccariello, G.; Cammaroto, G.; De Vito, A.; et al. Risk factors for obstructive sleep apnea syndrome in children: State of the art. *Int. J. Environ. Res. Public Health* **2019**, *16*, 3235. [CrossRef]
31. Tan, Y.H.; How, C.H.; Chan, Y.H.; Teoh, O.H. Approach to the snoring child. *Singap. Med. J.* **2020**, *61*, 170–175. [CrossRef]
32. Papaioannou, G.; Kambas, I.; Tsaoussoglou, M.; Panaghiotopoulou-Gartagani, P.; Chrousos, G.; Kaditis, A.G. Age-dependent changes in the size of adenotonsillar tissue in childhood: Implications for sleep-disordered breathing. *J. Pediatr.* **2013**, *162*, 269–274.e4. [CrossRef] [PubMed]

Disclaimer/Publisher's Note: The statements, opinions and data contained in all publications are solely those of the individual author(s) and contributor(s) and not of MDPI and/or the editor(s). MDPI and/or the editor(s) disclaim responsibility for any injury to people or property resulting from any ideas, methods, instructions or products referred to in the content.

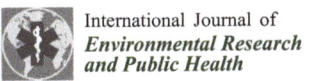

Viewpoint

Use of Irrigation Device for Duct Dilatation during Sialendoscopy

Giulio Pagliuca [1], Veronica Clemenzi [2,*], Andrea Stolfa [2], Salvatore Martellucci [1], Antonio Greco [2], Marco de Vincentiis [3] and Andrea Gallo [1,2]

1. Otolaryngology University Unit, Santa Maria Goretti Hospital, 04100 Latina, Italy
2. Department of Sensorial Organs, ENT Section, "Sapienza" University of Rome, 04100 Rome, Italy
3. Department of Oral and Maxillofacial Sciences, "Sapienza" University of Rome, 00161 Rome, Italy
* Correspondence: veronica.clemenzi@gmail.com; Tel.: +39-3203020207

Abstract: Background: Continuous irrigation of the duct with isotonic saline is one of the fundamental stages of a successful sialendoscopic procedure. It allows for an adequate luminal distension for the removal of debris and mucous plugs and for the conservative treatment of strictures. This procedure, which commonly involves the use of a medical syringe, can be laborious, and it is often necessary to interrupt irrigation during surgery due to the high resistance to saline. Setting: Academic university hospital. Method: We propose the use of an irrigation device which consists of a high-pressure syringe barrel, an ergonomic piston handle, and a gauge used to monitor the inflation and deflation of balloon catheters. The system allows for a simple and safe dilation, ensuring good visualization of the salivary duct lumen during sialendoscopy. Conclusions: The irrigation system described can be widely used to perform a diagnostic or interventional sialendoscopy more effectively than with a typical manual irrigation procedure.

Keywords: salivary gland; sialendoscopy; irrigation device; salivary duct

1. Introduction

Sialendoscopy, a minimally invasive procedure first mentioned by Kats in 1991, represents a continually expanding field and is becoming the preferred technique for diagnosing and managing salivary gland obstruction [1–3]. The continuous irrigation of the duct is one of the cardinal points of an effective sialendoscopic procedure. Irrigation with isotonic saline solution is necessary to overcome the sphincter-like contractile mechanism that keeps the duct in a collapsed state and allows an adequate luminal distension so that intraductal structures and pathologic changes of the duct can be clearly visualized. Irrigation also plays a pivotal therapeutic role, allowing for the removal of debris and mucous plugs from the ductal system and the conservative treatment of strictures, solving alone many of the most common obstructive conditions of the salivary glands [4]. Most surgeons opt for a manual irrigation process using a common medical syringe. This procedure can be laborious, and it is often necessary to interrupt irrigation during surgery due to the high resistance to saline. In this paper, we propose the use of an irrigation device that allows for the performance of a simple and safe dilation, ensuring good visualization of the salivary duct lumen during sialendoscopy.

2. Materials and Methods

During minimally invasive balloon dilation procedures, balloon inflation devices are widely used to inflate the balloon with fluid, monitor the pressure in the balloon during the procedure, and deflate the balloon after dilation. In ENT surgery, these devices are used mainly to dilate obstructed sinus ostia during sinuplasty in patients suffering from sinusitis, or to perform a Eustachian tube (ET) dilation to treat obstructive ET dysfunction, or during subglottic stenosis balloon dilation.

In this paper, we describe our experience with a balloon inflation device adapted to perform a constant irrigation of the salivary duct during sialendoscopy. Any patient showing an obstructive or inflammatory disease of the salivary glands could benefit from sialendoscopy performed with this new irrigation system. In our daily surgical practice, we use this device for irrigation on all patients undergoing sialendoscopy, regardless of the cause that generates the symptomatology.

The device (Figure 1) consists of a high-pressure syringe barrel, an ergonomic piston handle, and a gauge used to monitor the inflation and deflation of balloon catheters (Disposable Inflation Device, Cook Medical, AL, USA). In order to perform an adequate and constant dilation of the salivary glands, this device is connected with the irrigation channel of the sialendoscope and to a saline solution bottle through a three-way stop-cock (Figure 2). The stop-cock is positioned to allow the saline solution to flow from the bottle to the syringe of the device, which can be filled with 20 cc of solution (Figure 3a). The procedure is performed using an all-in-one Erlangen-type sialendoscope (Karl Storz, Tuttlingen, Germany) which are 1.1 mm in diameter for diagnostic and 1.3 or 1.6 mm for interventional sialendoscopy. Once the syringe of saline is filled, the device is locked, and the three-way stop-cock is rotated to allow the fluid to pass from the syringe to the sialendoscope (Figure 3b). The grip on the piston handle must be rotated clockwise to push the saline to the sialendoscope in order to increase the pressure in the ductal system until reaching the desired value. A gauge is used to monitor the pressure of saline in the salivary ducts. As a portion of the saline flows through the ductal orifice between the endoscope and the ductal walls and a portion is absorbed by the gland, the piston handle is rotated slowly and steadily to avoid the gradual decrease of the pressure in the ductal system. Turning the grip on the piston handle counterclockwise will decrease the pressure in the ducts. Once the saline solution in the syringe is depleted, the procedure can then be easily repeated, if needed.

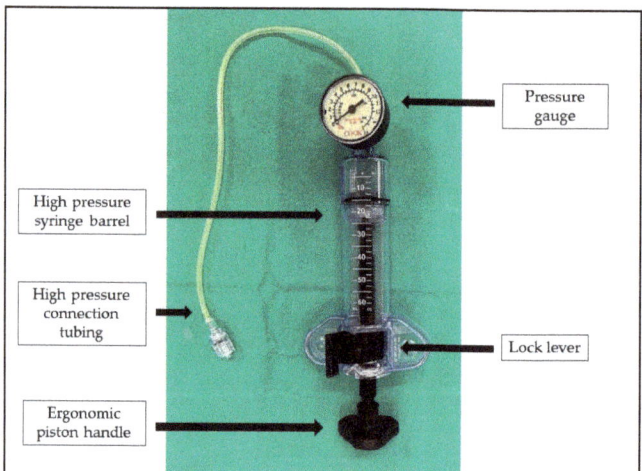

Figure 1. The irrigation device consists of a high-pressure syringe barrel, a lock lever, an ergonomic piston handle, a gauge used to monitor the inflation and deflation of balloon catheters, and connection tubing.

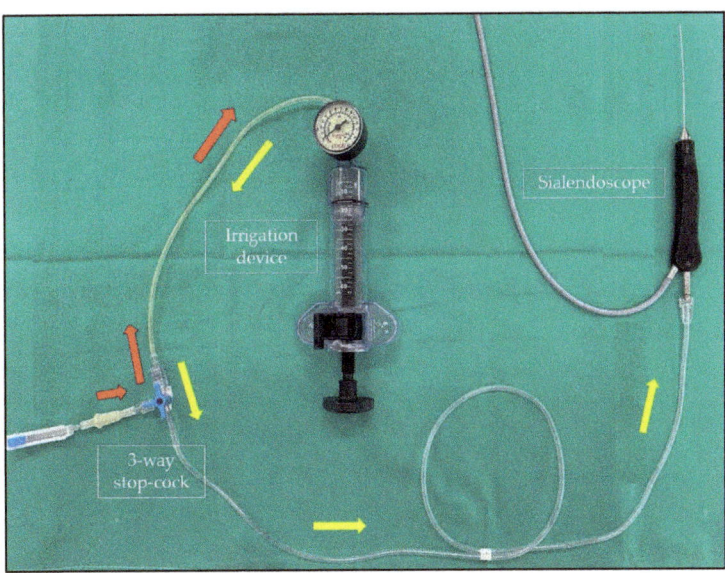

Figure 2. The irrigation device is connected with the irrigation channel of the sialendoscope and a saline solution bottle through a three-way stop-cock. Red arrows: saline solution is drawn into the syringe through the three-way stop-cock. Yellow arrows: saline solution is pushed into the sialendoscope through the three-way stop-cock under pressure control to perform an adequate duct dilatation.

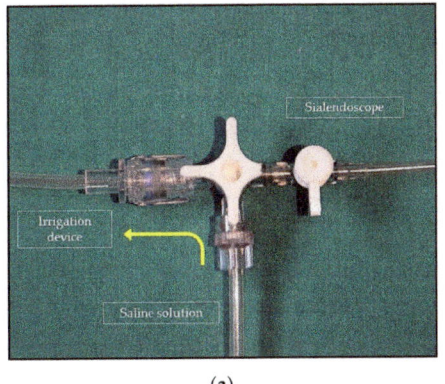
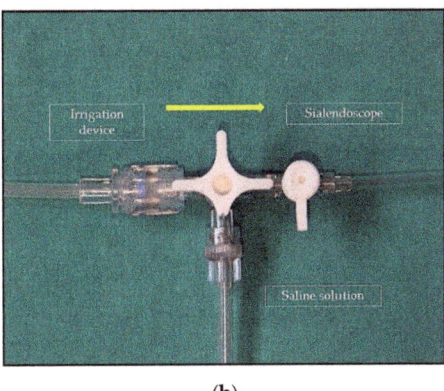

(a)   (b)

Figure 3. (a) The three-way stop-cock is positioned so as to allow saline to flow from the bottle to the syringe of the device, which can be filled with 20 cc of solution. (b) Once the syringe is filled with saline, the device is locked and the three-way stop-cock is rotated to allow fluid to pass from the syringe to the sialendoscope (b). The yellow arrows indicate the direction of the saline solution.

3. Discussion

Sialendoscopy is a procedure for the diagnosis and treatment of salivary obstructive and inflammatory diseases [5–8]. It can be performed under local or general anesthesia depending on the level of difficulty of the individual case. Continuous rinsing of the duct during the procedure is necessary to achieve its dilatation and consequently an adequate visualization of the lumen to allow the advancement of the scope into the duct system [9]. Irrigation allows us not only to obtain an effective dilation of the duct during endoscopy but also to treat some obstructive sialadenitis. The opportunity for administering drugs, such as corticosteroid preparations, directly into the ductal system provides an interesting point of access for salivary inflammatory disease therapy in adults and children [10–13]. Furthermore, the treatment of juvenile recurrent parotitis is based on dilation of the Stensen duct, and it is often performed using strong saline solution irrigation [14]. Continuous washing with a saline solution allows for the removal of mucous plugs from the lumen ducts, while the hydrostatic pressure on the ductal system can be considered a useful method to treat the strictures, especially in the case of multiple stenoses (often observed as a result of radioiodine therapy), when the use of a sialoballoon or of the sialendoscope itself does not allow the dilation of the whole stenotic tract [15]. In these cases, however, it is necessary to achieve and maintain an adequate pressure value during the surgical procedure to obtain a durable dilation and an effective washing of the ducts. Most surgeons opt for a manual irrigation performed by an assistant using a typical medical syringe connected to the irrigation channel of the sialendoscope through a connecting tube. The information found in the literature indicates that the intraductal pressures achieved with a 20 mL syringe are greater than or equal to those obtained with a 10 mL syringe, but in the former case, the second operator applies a much higher force when working with a larger syringe, without direct control of the pressure inside the salivary duct system [16]. While it is widely used, this procedure can be laborious, and it is often necessary to interrupt irrigation during surgery because of the high resistance to saline solution. Additionally, the pressure achievable by manual irrigation may not be sufficient to ensure an effective and permanent dilation of the stenoses.

This paper presents a safe, less laborious, and simple method to perform efficient dilation of the salivary glands ducts during sialendoscopy using an adapted Cook Balloon Inflation Device. The patients were fully informed during the consent procedure of the risks associated regarding the off-label use of this medical device, and their informed consents were recorded. This revised irrigation system allows us to reach the desired pressure value and maintain it for as long as necessary, permitting optimal visualization of the duct and an effective progression of the endoscope into the ductal system. The saline pressure provides a radial force equally distributed in all directions in the ductal system and allows for the dilation of an entire stenotic tract, reaching a theoretical maximum pressure of 15 atmospheres on the ductal walls. The use of this device could allow the assisting nurse to completely replace the second operator in maneuvering the device during sialendoscopy.

During our clinical experience, no complications resulting from the use of this device were observed. The device is currently used without contraindications for all the patients who undergo sialendoscopic procedure.

4. Conclusions

The irrigation system described in this paper has proven to be more effective than a typical, often laborious, manual irrigation and can be widely used to perform dilation of the ducts of salivary glands during diagnostic or interventional sialendoscopy.

- During sialendoscopy, a continuous rinsing of the duct is necessary to achieve dilatation of the duct and an adequate visualization of the lumen.
- Manual irrigation with medical syringe is sometimes tiring and unwarranted.
- The adapted balloon inflation device permits a non-laborious duct irrigation and dilation under pression control in any patient who undergoes sialendoscopy.

Funding: This research received no external funding.

Informed Consent Statement: Informed consent was obtained from all subjects involved in the study.

Data Availability Statement: Not applicable.

Conflicts of Interest: The authors declare no conflict of interest.

References

1. Katz, P. Endoscopie des glandes salivaires [Endoscopy of the salivary glands]. *Ann. Radiol.* **1991**, *34*, 110–113. (In French) [PubMed]
2. Gillespie, M.B.; Intaphan, J.; Nguyen, S.A. Endoscopic-assisted management of chronic sialadenitis. *Head Neck.* **2011**, *33*, 1346–1351. [CrossRef] [PubMed]
3. Gallo, A.; Benazzo, M.; Capaccio, P.; De Campora, L.; De Vincentiis, M.; Fusconi, M.; Martellucci, S.; Paludetti, G.; Pasquini, E.; Puxeddu, R.; et al. Sialoendoscopy: State of the art, challenges and further perspectives. Round Table, 101(st) SIO National Congress, Catania 2014. *Acta Otorhinolaryngol. Ital.* **2015**, *35*, 217–233. [PubMed]
4. Koch, M.; Zenk, J.; Bozzato, A.; Bumm, K.; Iro, H. Sialoscopy in cases of unclear swelling of the major salivary glands. *Otolaryngol. Head Neck Surg.* **2005**, *133*, 863–868. [CrossRef] [PubMed]
5. Colella, G.; Lo Giudice, G.; De Luca, R.; Troiano, A.; Lo Faro, C.; Santillo, V.; Tartaro, G. Interventional sialendoscopy in parotidomegaly related to eating disorders. *J. Eat. Disord.* **2021**, *9*, 25. [CrossRef] [PubMed]
6. Lo Giudice, G.; Marra, P.M.; Colella, C.; Itro, A.; Tartaro, G.; Colella, G. Salivary Gland Disorders in Pediatric Patients: A 20 Years' Experience. *Appl. Sci.* **2022**, *12*, 1999. [CrossRef]
7. Fusconi, M.; Meliante, P.G.; Pagliuca, G.; Greco, A.; de Vincentiis, M.; Polimeni, A.; Musy, I.; Candelori, F.; Gallo, A. Interpretation of the mucous plug through sialendoscopy. *Oral Dis.* **2022**, *28*, 384–389. [CrossRef] [PubMed]
8. Marchal, F.; Dulguerov, P.; Becker, M.; Barki, G.; Disant, F.; Lehmann, W. Submandibular diagnostic and interventional sialendoscopy: New procedure for ductal disorders. *Ann. Otol. Rhinol. Laryngol.* **2002**, *111*, 27–35. [CrossRef] [PubMed]
9. Nahlieli, O.; Baruchin, A.M. Long-term experience with endoscopic diagnosis and treatment of salivary gland inflammatory diseases. *Laryngoscope* **2000**, *110*, 988–993. [CrossRef] [PubMed]
10. Gallo, A.; Capaccio, P.; Benazzo, M.; De Campora, L.; De Vincentiis, M.; Farneti, P.; Fusconi, M.; Gaffuri, M.; Lo Russo, F.; Martellucci, S.; et al. Outcomes of interventional sialendoscopy for obstructive salivary gland disorders: An Italian multicentre study. *Acta Otorhinolaryngol. Ital.* **2016**, *36*, 479–485. [CrossRef] [PubMed]
11. Gallo, A.; Martellucci, S.; Fusconi, M.; Pagliuca, G.; Greco, A.; De Virgilio, A.; De Vincentiis, M. Sialendoscopic management of autoimmune sialadenitis: A review of literature. *Acta Otorhinolaryngol. Ital.* **2017**, *37*, 148–154. [CrossRef] [PubMed]
12. Nahlieli, O.; Nazarian, Y. Sialadenitis following radioiodine therapy—A new diagnostic and treatment modality. *Oral Dis.* **2006**, *12*, 476–479. [CrossRef] [PubMed]
13. Gallo, A.; Clemenzi, V.; Stolfa, A.; Pagliuca, G.; Benedetti, F.M.N.; Caporale, C.; del Giudice, A.M.; Maino, T.; de Robertis, V.; Cariti, F.; et al. The secretory senescence of the oro-pharyngo-laryngeal tract. *J. Gerontol. Geriatr.* **2020**, *68*, 69–76. [CrossRef]
14. Shacham, R.; Droma, E.B.; London, D.; Bar, T.; Nahlieli, O. Long-term experience with endoscopic diagnosis and treatment of juvenile recurrent parotitis. *J. Oral Maxillofac. Surg.* **2009**, *67*, 162–167. [CrossRef] [PubMed]
15. Ardekian, L.; Shamir, D.; Trabelsi, M.; Peled, M. Chronic obstructive parotitis due to strictures of Stenson's duct–our treatment experience with sialoendoscopy. *J. Oral Maxillofac. Surg.* **2010**, *68*, 83–87. [CrossRef] [PubMed]
16. Luers, J.C.; Ortmann, M.; Beutner, D.; Hüttenbrink, K.B. Intraductal pressure during sialendoscopy. *J. Laryngol. Otol.* **2014**, *128*, 897–901. [CrossRef] [PubMed]

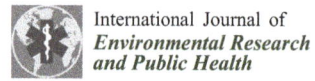

Article

Hearing Problems in Indonesia: Attention to Hypertensive Adults

Melysa Fitriana [1,2] and Chyi-Huey Bai [1,3,4,*]

1. International Master/Ph.D. Program in Medicine, College of Medicine, Taipei Medical University, Taipei 11031, Taiwan; melysa.fitriana@mail.ugm.ac.id
2. Otorhinolaryngology Head and Neck Surgery Department, Faculty of Medicine, Public Health and Nursing, Universitas Gadjah Mada, Yogyakarta 55281, Indonesia
3. School of Public Health, College of Public Health, Taipei Medical University, Taipei 11031, Taiwan
4. Department of Public Health, College of Medicine, Taipei Medical University, Taipei 11031, Taiwan
* Correspondence: baich@tmu.edu.tw; Tel.: +886-(2)-2736-1661 (ext. 6510)

Abstract: Known as a silent disability, hearing loss is one of the major health burdens worldwide. Evidence implies that those suffering from hypertension can experience hearing disturbances. Self-reporting of hearing problems and self-reporting of hypertension may be useful in providing an alarm for detecting hearing problems. However, in the Indonesian population, this matter has not been properly reported. The aim of this study was to explore the prevalence of hearing problems and their relationships with other demographic factors. In total, 28,297 respondents of productive age from the Indonesian Family Life Survey 5th wave were assessed. A questionnaire and physical examination data were included in this survey. Self-reported hearing problems and their predictors were analyzed using univariate and multivariate logistic regressions. Hypertension awareness was a significant predictor of having a hearing problem (odds ratio (OR) [95% confidence interval (CI)], p value: 2.715 [1.948~3.785], <0.001). Having a general check-up was also crucial for detecting hearing problems (2.192 [1.54~3.121], <0.001). There was a significant link between hearing problems and early adults who have isolated systolic hypertension. Hypertension awareness and having a general check-up had predictive value for detecting hearing problems in adults in the age range of 26~35 years. Therefore, public health strategies for hearing loss prevention might target this group by detecting and treating hypertension.

Keywords: hearing problem; hypertension; adult; IFLS

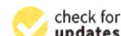

Citation: Fitriana, M.; Bai, C.-H. Hearing Problems in Indonesia: Attention to Hypertensive Adults. *Int. J. Environ. Res. Public Health* **2022**, *19*, 9222. https://doi.org/10.3390/ijerph19159222

Academic Editors: Paul B. Tchounwou, Francesco Gazia, Bruno Galletti, Gay-Escoda Cosme, Francesco Ciodaro and Rocco Bruno

Received: 26 May 2022
Accepted: 26 July 2022
Published: 28 July 2022

Publisher's Note: MDPI stays neutral with regard to jurisdictional claims in published maps and institutional affiliations.

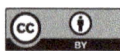

Copyright: © 2022 by the authors. Licensee MDPI, Basel, Switzerland. This article is an open access article distributed under the terms and conditions of the Creative Commons Attribution (CC BY) license (https://creativecommons.org/licenses/by/4.0/).

1. Introduction

The sense of hearing is important for humans to communicate with other people and also to interact within the community. With advancements in hearing technologies in the past few decades, identifying and diagnosing hearing impairment can be completed in many settings. Around 360 million people (over 5%) all over the world live with this disability (disabling hearing loss), which makes hearing loss a factor that is responsible for years lived with a disability [1,2]. Among the six World Health Organization (WHO) regions, the highest prevalence of hearing loss is in the western Pacific region (with 136.5 million people), followed by Southeast Asia (with 109.5 million people) [3].

Loss of productivity and social isolation might result from communication difficulties caused by hearing impairment [4,5]. A systematic review of the global burden of disease from 1990 to 2019 revealed that 1.57 billion people worldwide suffered from hearing impairment in 2019. An estimate was made that by 2050, there will be 2.45 billion people with a hearing decline (one of every four people), an increase of 56.1% from 2019 [6]. Although there are approximately 40 million American adults who suffer from various degrees of hearing impairment, there are gaps between self-reported hearing loss and people who receive a hearing test and treatment for hearing impairment [7]. Patients who have self-recognized hearing disturbances should undergo a hearing evaluation by a medical professional such as an ear, nose, and throat (ENT) doctor or audiologist [8].

Based on the National Health and Nutrition Examination Survey in 2015–2018, the prevalence of high blood pressure increases with age, at 28.2% among 20~44 year olds, at 60.1% in 45~64 year olds, and 77% among those older than 65 years [9]. On the other hand, low- and middle-income countries (LMICs; with 1.04 billion people accounting for 31.5% of the world's population) had a higher prevalence of hypertension compared to high-income countries (HICs; with 349 million people or 28.5% of the world's population) [10,11]. Unfortunately, in spite of the increasing hypertension prevalence, hypertension awareness and treatment in LMICs are still low, including in Indonesia, which had treatment rates of less than 25% of women, as well as men which less than 20% [10,12]. For several decades (1990~2019) the hypertension burden has increased in young adults [13]. In Asian populations, the prevalence of isolated systolic hypertension (ISH) has increased due to special epidemiological characteristics and risk factors and greater susceptibility to ISH [14]. Likewise, a previous study also implied that systolic blood pressure (SBP) levels are considered a crucial factor in preventing and treating hypertension [15].

Epidemiological studies of hearing loss and hypertension as vascular risk factors supported the fact that there is a significant link between the two [16,17]. However, the molecular mechanism behind this association is still under investigation, and it could be due to vascular injury [18,19]. A recent cohort study investigating hearing loss and blood pressure was conducted in Japanese adults, and those findings suggested that a higher SBP condition was a significant risk factor for hearing loss at 1 kHz [3]. A long time ago, the crucial role of SBP was already mentioned in the Framingham Heart study which determined that SBP had a larger capacity in the future risk of cardiovascular disease than diastolic blood pressure (DBP) [20,21].

In this study, our main aim was to investigate the prevalence of hearing problems of various ages and blood pressure conditions. Later, we assessed the relationship between hearing problems and blood pressure based on subjects' age groups in an Indonesian population.

2. Materials and Methods

2.1. Study Population and Participants

The Indonesian Family Life Survey 5th wave (IFLS5) 2014 was used in this study. The IFLS5 is a cross-sectional national survey that focuses on health and socioeconomic fields and was conducted from late 2014 to early 2015. Data were collected by assessing individual respondents, their households, and community levels. The IFLS survey is a longitudinal survey designed to provide public use data to investigate behaviors and outputs, and to the present, there have been five waves of surveys that are available on their website. In the first wave in 1993, 20 households from urban regions and 30 households from rural regions in 13 of 27 provinces in Indonesia were selected by random sampling. IFLS5 was chosen as the data source in this study because it has the most complete data compared to previous waves. A well-designed structured questionnaire was administered through in-person interviews by well-trained interviewers. A physical examination including blood pressure, body height, and body weight was also conducted [22]. Our study population included all of the participants of the IFLS5, and the sample consisted of those who met the inclusion and exclusion criteria. The inclusion criterion was an age range of 15~64 years, and exclusion criteria were missing data of gender, blood pressure, height, or weight. Ultimately, 28,297 participants were enrolled as seen in Figure 1.

2.2. Age Categories

Respondents' ages ranged from 15 to 64 years, which is considered productive age in the Indonesian population. Furthermore, age was divided into four groups based on Indonesia Ministry of Health criteria: (1) 15~25 years as adolescence, (2) 26~35 years old as early adulthood, (3) 36~45 years old as late adulthood, and (4) 46~64 years old as elderly.

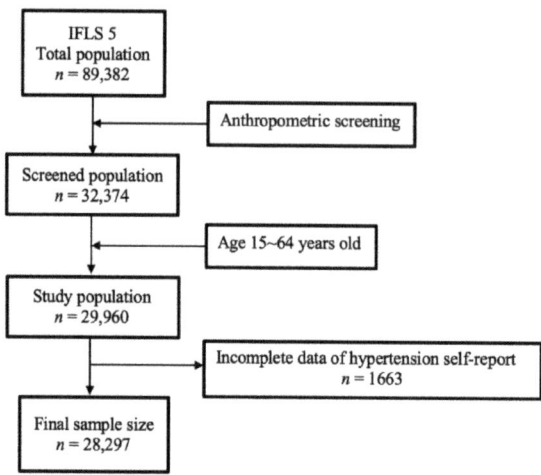

Figure 1. Sample screening process.

2.3. Blood Pressure

Blood pressure was measured three times by trained interviewers using an Omron meter (HEM-7203) on alternate arms in a seated position. A normal size cuff was generally used, while larger cuffs were also provided if needed. Averages of the systole and diastole data were determined. Later, blood pressure data were classified using the modified-American Heart Association (AHA) 2017 and Indonesian Society of Hypertension (INASH) 2019 criteria. AHA 2017 [23] criteria for blood pressure were modified into three groups: (1) normal blood pressure (systole < 120 mmHg and diastole < 80 mmHg), (2) elevated blood pressure (systole 120~129 mmHg and diastole < 80 mmHg) and (3) hypertension (systole ≥ 130 mmHg and diastole ≥ 80 mmHg).

To evaluate specific cases of ISH, additional criteria of the INASH 2019 with modifications were also added. The modified INASH version only has two groups which are non-ISH (a combination of optimal, normal, high normal, and grades 1, 2, and 3 hypertensive groups) and ISH. Originally, the INASH criteria had several groups of blood pressure, which included (1) optimal (systole < 120 mmHg and diastole < 80 mmHg), (2) normal (systole 120~129 mmHg and diastole 80~84 mmHg), (3) high-normal (systole 130~139 mmHg and diastole 85~89 mmHg), (4) grade 1 hypertension (systole 140~159 mmHg and diastole 90~99 mmHg), (5) grade 2 hypertension (systole 160~179 mmHg and diastole 100~109 mmHg), (6) grade 3 hypertension (systole ≥ 180 mmHg and diastole ≥ 110 mmHg), and (7) ISH (systole ≥ 140 mmHg and diastole < 90 mmHg) [24].

2.4. Hearing Problems-Self Reported

Hearing problems were assessed by answering a question about hearing problems (have you been diagnosed with a hearing problem by a doctor, paramedic, nurse, or midwife?).

2.5. Covariates

Covariates consisted of hypertension-self reported, hypertension medication, body mass index (BMI), educational level, occupation, general check-ups, outpatient care, insurance coverage, and hearing aid usage. Information on hypertension self-reported was collected by answering a question about a diagnosis of hypertension (yes or no). Likewise, hypertension medication was reported by answering a question about a history of undergoing hypertension treatment (yes or no).

The BMI was calculated using height divided by weight squared (kg/m^2) from physical measurements. A Seca model 213 plastic height board was used to measure height to the closest millimeter. A Camry model EB1003 scale was used to calculate body weight to the nearest 0.1 kg. Finally, the BMI was categorized into four groups based on Indonesia Ministry of Health criteria, which are (1) underweight (BMI < 18.5 kg/m^2), (2) normal (BMI 18.5~25 kg/m^2), (3) overweight–mild (BMI 25.1~27 kg/m^2), and (4) overweight–severe (BMI > 27 kg/m^2).

Educational data were grouped into three categories, including (1) no schooling, (2) senior high school or lower (graduated), and (3) above senior high school (graduated). The occupational status was noted with questions about whether the respondent had worked within the past year and had the same job for more than 5 years. General check-ups, outpatient care, insurance, and hearing aid usage were recorded by answering questions of having had a general check-up in the last 5 years, having had outpatient care in the last 4 weeks, having a health card, and ever having to wear a hearing aid (all yes or no), respectively.

2.6. Statistical Analysis

Descriptive analyses were used to show characteristics of study participants. The frequency, percentage, chi-squared test, or Fisher exact test for categorical data and the mean, standard deviation (SD), and Student's *t*-test for continuous data were used. The odds ratio (OR), 95% confidence interval (CI), and *p* value were calculated using univariate and multivariate logistic regressions. A subgroup analysis was carried out by gender. All statistical analyses were performed with SPSS software vers. 26 (IBM, Armonk, NY, USA). A *p* value of <0.05 was accepted as statistically significant.

3. Results

3.1. Characteristics of the Population

Of the 28,297 total individuals (age (mean ± SD): 35.29 ± 12.78 years for men and 35.01 ± 12.79 years for women) from the Indonesian population, 220 people had hearing problems (for a prevalence of 7.8 per 1000 persons). The prevalence of self-reported hearing problems in those aged 15~25, 26~35, 36~45, and 46~64 years was 0.48, 0.48, 0.85, and 1.4 per 1000 persons, respectively. Thus, the prevalence of hearing problems increased with age. In addition, hearing problems were more prevalent among subjects with elevated blood pressure or hypertension, those with isolated hypertension, those taking antihypertensive drugs, those with self-reported hypertension, those employed, those with a general check-up in the past 5 years, and those with outpatient treatment in the last 4 weeks. Among those who were experiencing hearing problems, 51.4% were male and 48.6% were female, but none of them were using a hearing aid.

Overall, the hypertensive group comprised a majority of the population according to AHA 2017 criteria which was 12,843 participants. The prevalence of hypertension based on AHA 2017 criteria was 45.38 per 100 persons in this Indonesian population aged 15~64 years. Hypertension was not significantly correlated with hearing problems (p = 0.093). According to the criterion of the INASH 2019, the prevalence of isolated systolic hypertension was 6.3 per 100 persons.

Those participants with hearing problems had a significantly (p = 0.048) higher proportion of isolated hypertension (9.5%) than those without such problems (6.3%). Surprisingly, among those with hearing problems, only 26.8% were aware that they had hypertension and 7.7% were treating it with hypertension medication.

There were correlations of hearing problems with being employed (p = 0.007), having had a recent general check-up (p < 0.001), and having had recent outpatient care (p = 0.003). Although the prevalence of hearing problems in the worker group at 77.3% was higher than in the non-worker group, the number of hearing problems was higher in the group who had had a general check-up in the past 5 years and those who had had outpatient care in the past 4 weeks.

Such positive correlations were not found for the BMI, educational level, or insurance ownership (Table 1).

Table 1. Distributions of demographic data based on hearing problems.

	N Total	Prevalence of Hearing Problems (%)	Hearing Problems				X^2	p Value
			No		Yes			
			n	%	n	%		
Age group (years)								
15–25	7452	0.48	7416	26.4	36	16.4		
26–35	8179	0.48	8139	29	40	18.2	50.815	0.000
36–45	6193	0.85	6140	21.9	53	24.1		
46–64	6473	1.4	6382	22.7	91	41.4		
Gender								
Male	13,147	0.85	13,034	46.4	113	51.4	2.14	0.143
Female	15,150	0.7	15,043	53.6	107	48.6		
Blood pressure								
AHA 2017								
Normal	11,153	0.63	11,082	39.5	71	32.3		
Elevated	4301	0.86	4264	15.2	37	16.8	4.741	0.093
Hypertensive	12,843	0.87	12,731	45.3	112	50.9		
INAHS 2019								
Non-isolated systolic hypertensive	26,510	0.75	26,311	93.7	199	90.5	3.911	0.048
Isolated systolic hypertensive	1787	1.17	1766	6.3	21	9.5		
Hypertension medication								
Yes	581	2.92	465	2	17	7.7	35.49	0.000
No	27,716	0.73	27,513	98	203	92.3		
Self-reported hypertension								
Yes	3004	1.96	2945	10.5	59	26.8	61.34	0.000
No	25,293	0.63	25,132	89.5	161	73.2		
Body mass index group								
Underweight	3366	0.38	3353	11.9	13	5.9		
Normal	15,856	0.83	15,723	56	133	60.5	7.76	0.053
Overweight–mild	3543	0.79	3515	12.5	28	12.7		
Overweight–severe	5532	0.83	5486	19.5	46	20.9		
Education								
No schooling	7920	0.77	7859	28	61	27.7		
Senior high school or lower	17,664	0.75	17,532	62.4	132	60	1.88	0.39
Above senior high school	2713	0.99	2686	9.6	27	12.3		
Occupation								
Working	19,474	0.87	19,304	68.8	170	77.3	7.38	0.007
Not working	8823	0.57	8773	31.2	50	22.7		
General check-up								
Yes	2514	1.63	2473	8.8	41	18.6	26.05	0.000
No	25,783	0.69	25,604	91.2	179	81.4		
Outpatient care								
Yes	5015	1.12	4959	17.7	56	25.5	9.09	0.003
No	23,282	0.7	23,118	82.3	164	74.5		
Insurance ownership								
Yes	14,183	0.8	14,069	50.1	114	51.8	0.25	0.613
No	14,114	0.75	14,008	49.9	106	48.2		
Hearing aid usage								
Yes	19	0	19	0.1	0	0	0.15	0.7
No	28,278	0.78	28,058	99.9	220	100		

AHA, American Heart Association; INASH, Indonesian Society of Hypertension.

3.2. Univariate Analysis of Hearing Problems with Demographic Data

Table 2 shows relationships between self-reported hearing problems as the dependent variable and other independent variables. There were significant associations (all $p < 0.05$) between hearing problems and age group, with the strongest protective effects in those aged 46–64 years. Otherwise, gender was not correlated with hearing problems ($p = 0.144$).

Table 2. Univariate logistic regression of hearing problems and demographic data.

Predictor	Coef.	SE Coef.	Wald	p	Odds Ratio	95% CI Lower	95% CI Upper
Age group (years)							
15~25	−0.576	0.217	7.057	0.008	0.562	0.368	0.86
26~35	−0.563	0.21	7.185	0.007	0.569	0.377	0.859
36~45					1.0		
46~64	0.502	0.174	8.348	0.004	1.652	1.175	2.322
Gender							
Male	0.198	0.135	2.136	0.144	1.219	0.935	1.589
Female					1.0		
Blood pressure							
AHA 2017							
Normal					1.0		
Elevated	0.303	0.204	2.221	0.136	1.354	0.909	2.018
Hypertensive	0.317	0.152	4.338	0.037	1.373	1.019	1.851
INAHS 2019							
Non-isolated systolic hypertensive					1.0		
Isolated systolic hypertensive	0.452	0.231	3.845	0.05	1.572	1.0	2.471
Hypertension medication							
Yes	1.407	0.256	30.212	0.000	4.085	2.473	6.748
No					1.0		
Self-reported hypertension							
Yes	1.140	0.153	55.225	0.000	3.127	2.315	4.224
No					1.0		
Body mass index group							
Underweight	−0.771	0.315	6.001	0.014	0.462	0.249	0.857
Normal	0.009	0.172	0.003	0.959	1.009	0.72	1.413
Overweight–mild	−0.051	0.241	0.43	0.831	0.95	0.593	1.523
Overweight–severe					1.0		
Educational level							
No schooling	−0.259	0.232	1.24	0.266	0.772	0.49	1.217
Senior high school or lower	−0.289	0.212	1.854	0.173	0.749	0.494	1.135
Above senior high school					1.0		
Occupation							
Working	0.435	0.161	7.269	0.007	1.545	1.126	2.12
Not working					1.0		
General check-up							
Yes	0.864	0.174	24.511	0.000	2.371	1.685	3.338
No					1.0		
Outpatient care							
Yes	0.465	0.156	8.931	0.003	1.592	1.174	2.159
No					1.0		
Insurance ownership							
Yes	0.068	0.135	0.255	0.614	1.071	0.821	1.396
No					1.0		

AHA, American Heart Association; INASH, Indonesian Society of Hypertension; Coef., coefficient; SE, standard error; CI, confidence interval.

Based on all criteria for hypertension by AHA and INASH, significant risks were shown in the hypertension group (OR [95% CI], p value; 1.373 [0.019~1.851], 0.037) and in the isolated hypertension group (1.572 [1.0~2.471], 0.05) compared to the reference group. This shows that having hearing problems was related to a hypertensive condition. Likewise, self-reported hypertension (3.127 [2.315~4.224] <0.001) and related treatment (4.085 [2.473~6.748], <0.001) had large risk effects on hearing problems.

A general check-up (2.371 [1.685~3.338], <0.001) and outpatient care (1.592 [1.174~2.159], 0.003) among participants had significant risks for the occurrence of hearing problems. In addition, the underweight group based on the BMI had a significant protective effect against hearing problems (0.462 [0.249~0.857], 0.014) compared to the overweight group.

Having a job seems to be related to hearing problems (1.545 [1.126~2.12], 0.007) compared to not having a job. Nevertheless, there was no relationship between hearing problems and educational level or insurance ownership (Table 2).

3.3. Association of Self-Reported Hypertension and General Check-Ups with Hearing Problems in Adults

Since the age and blood pressure categories were highly correlated with hearing problems, the combined effect of age group and blood pressure categories (hereafter referred to as the interaction of age*blood pressure) with hearing problems was next assessed. Subsequently, several models were developed to predict having hearing problems based on univariate $p < 0.05$ of covariates (Table 3). Compared to the full model, the general check-up and outpatient care variables were excluded in model 1. On the other hand, self-reported hypertension and outpatient care variables were excluded in model 2. In model 3 (the full model), compared to 36~45-year-old adults with normal blood pressure, hearing problems were negatively associated with participants who had elevated blood pressure in early adults (0.398 [0.165~0.959], 0.04) and the elderly (0.325 [0.11~0.961], 0.042), and were positively associated with participants who had elevated blood pressure in adolescents (2.165 [1.11~4.24], 0.023). In addition, significant positive relationships with hearing problems were found in subjects with both self-reported hypertension and having had a general check-up.

Table 3. Multivariate logistic regression analysis of hearing problems.

	Predictor	Model 1				Model 2				Full Model		
		p	Odds Ratio	95% CI Lower	95% CI Upper	p	Odds Ratio	95% CI Lower	95% CI Upper	p	Odds Ratio	95% CI Lower	95% CI Upper
	(Constant)	0.000	0.007			0.000	0.007			0.000	0.005		
	Age (years) * AHA category												
1	(15~25) * Normal BP	0.45	0.783	0.414	1.478	0.339	0.733	0.388	1.386	0.461	0.787	0.417	1.488
2	(15~25) * Elevated BP	0.335	0.648	0.268	1.567	0.288	0.619	0.256	1.499	0.325	0.642	0.265	1.552
3	(15~25) * Hypertension	0.036	0.391	0.162	0.941	0.041	0.399	0.166	0.961	0.04	0.398	0.165	0.959
4	(26~35) * Normal BP	0.1	0.584	0.308	1.108	0.084	0.568	0.3	1.078	0.103	0.587	0.309	1.114
5	(26~35) * Elevated BP	0.037	0.315	0.107	0.931	0.044	0.329	0.111	0.972	0.042	0.325	0.11	0.961
6	(26~35) * Hypertension	0.078	0.551	0.284	1.068	0.136	0.604	0.312	1.171	0.091	0.564	0.291	1.095
7	(36~45) * Normal BP		1.0				1.0				1.0		
8	(36~45) * Elevated BP	0.984	1.027	0.461	2.288	0.781	1.12	0.503	2.496	0.855	1.077	0.483	2.402
9	(36~45) * Hypertension	0.305	0.727	0.395	1.337	0.593	0.848	0.462	1.554	0.344	0.745	0.405	1.371
10	(46~64) * Normal BP	0.799	1.102	0.52	2.335	0.808	1.097	0.518	2.324	0.836	1.083	0.511	2.294
11	(46~64) * Elevated BP	0.019	2.23	1.144	4.346	0.012	2.36	1.212	4.593	0.023	2.165	1.11	4.224
12	(46~64) * Hypertension	0.562	1.174	0.683	2.016	0.094	1.568	0.926	2.654	0.562	1.174	0.683	2.018
	Gender	0.108	1.273	0.949	1.709	0.365	1.146	0.854	1.537	0.128	1.259	0.936	1.692
	Body mass index group												
	Underweight	0.115	0.592	0.309	1.136	0.101	0.58	0.303	1.112	0.164	0.63	0.328	1.208
	Normal	0.401	1.165	0.815	1.666	0.481	1.137	0.796	1.623	0.265	1.226	0.857	1.755
	Overweight–mild	0.936	0.981	0.61	1.577	0.848	0.954	0.594	1.535	0.974	0.992	0.617	1.596
	Overweight–severe		1.0				1.0				1.0		
	Self-reported hypertension	0.000	2.715	1.948	3.785					0.000	2.48	1.77	3.474
	General check-up					0.000	2.192	1.54	3.121	0.000	1.976	1.384	2.821
	Outpatient care									0.066	1.343	0.981	1.839
	Education												
	No schooling	0.157	0.712	0.444	1.14	0.49	0.844	0.521	1.366	0.487	0.843	0.521	1.364
	Senior high school or lower	0.266	0.788	0.517	1.199	0.586	0.888	0.58	1.361	0.604	0.893	0.583	1.369
	Above senior high school		1.0				1.0				1.0		
	Occupation	0.257	1.225	0.862	1.742	0.362	1.179	0.828	1.678	0.242	1.233	0.868	1.753
	Insurance ownership	0.631	1.067	0.818	1.393	0.651	1.063	0.815	1.388	0.685	1.057	0.809	1.379

AHA, American Heart Association; BP, Blood Pressure; CI, confidence interval; *, Combine effect of age and blood pressure groups.

Further analysis showed that self-reported hypertension seemed to be an important predictor for having hearing problems as seen in model 1 (2.715 [1.948~3.785], <0.001). In addition, as seen in model 2, having a general check-up was a significant predictor for hearing problem conditions (2.192 [1.54~3.121], <0.001). These findings illustrate that hypertension awareness and having a general check-up are important factors; however, after adjusting for such factors, elevated blood pressure was still important to prevent hearing problems in early adults (26~35 years of age) (Table 3).

3.4. Protective Value of Self-Reported Hypertension and a General Check-Up to Hearing Problems in Early Adults

There was also a combined effect of age and blood pressure categories in INASH-isolated systolic hypertension which were shown in Table 4 after adjustment for covariates (gender, BMI, hypertension self-reported, general check-up, outpatient care, educational level, occupation, and insurance ownership). Compared to subjects aged 36~45 years and those without isolated systolic hypertension, there was a significant protective effect against hearing problems in early adults (26~35 years of age) (0.6 [0.394~0.915], 0.0018). The risk of hearing problems was also seen in the aged group (46~64 years) compared to those aged 36~45 years without isolated systolic hypertension (Table 4).

Table 4. Combination effect of age and blood pressure criteria on hearing problems.

	Predictors	Coef.	SE Coef.	Wald	p	Odds Ratio	95% CI Lower	95% CI Upper
	Age (years) * INASH-isosysht							
1	(15~25) * Non-isosysht	−0.315	0.232	1.849	0.174	0.73	0.463	1.149
2	(15~25) * Isosysht	−16.398	2764.809	0.000	0.995	0.000	0.000	-
3	(26~35) * Non-isosysht	−0.511	0.215	5.641	0.018	0.6	0.394	0.915
4	(26~35) * Isosysht	−0.667	1.014	0.433	0.511	0.513	0.07	3.745
5	(36~45) * Non-isosysht					1.0		
6	(36~45) * Isosysht	−0.36	0.724	0.246	0.62	0.698	0.169	2.887
7	(46~64) * Non-isosysht	0.337	0.19	3.156	0.076	1.401	0.966	2.032
8	(46~64) * Isosysht	0.526	0.284	3.419	0.064	1.692	0.969	2.954

Adjusted for all predictors (gender, body mass index group, hypertension self-reported, general check-up, outpatient care, educational level, occupation, and insurance ownership). Coef., coefficient; SE, standard error; CI, confidence interval; AHA, American Heart Association; BP, blood pressure; INASH, Indonesian Society of Hypertension; Non-isosysht, non-isolated systolic hypertension; Isosysht, isolated systolic hypertension; *, Combine effect of age and blood pressure groups.

In addition, the subgroup analysis by gender had been performed. The result from the gender analysis showed insignificant results due to the small sample size in hearing problems (Tables S1 and S2).

4. Discussion

The study finding of a combined effect of age and blood pressure on hearing problems stresses the importance of the SBP condition in early adults (26~35 years of age) to prevent hearing problems. Hence, to eliminate the risk of hearing problems related to hypertension, public health professionals might target this population age range.

There was a slightly higher prevalence of hearing problems in men (51.4%) than in women (48.6%) in this study. Meanwhile, the global prevalence of hearing loss at moderate or higher levels among men is slightly higher than that of women, at 217 million (5.6%) and 211 million (5.5%), respectively [25]. Interestingly, a study conducted in 2017 showed that males were nearly two-fold more likely compared to women to have hearing impairment in populations ranging 20 to 69 years of age [26]. In contrast to a previous study in Japan, 46.7% of men and 53.2% of women had hearing impairment. Moreover, a higher risk of hearing problems occurred in both males and females with hypertension [27]. On the other hand, specifically in the male population, hypertension was positively related to hearing impairment at a prevalence ratio of 1.52 per 1000 persons with a 95% CI of 1.07~2.16 [17].

Study findings in a Canadian population showed that the prevalence of hearing problems (79%) was higher among adults with hypertension [27]. Additionally, the highest rate of hearing loss was in the group 60~69 years old [26]. Both of those findings support our finding that there was an increasing prevalence rate with age. In addition, a previous study revealed that age is known to be the strongest predictor of hearing impairment in adults (range 20~69 years old) [26]. Likewise, we found that each age group was positively associated with hearing problems ($p < 0.05$).

Based on a modified AHA 2017 grouping of blood pressure, we also found that the hypertensive group was associated with hearing problems ($p = 0.037$) as well as the modified–isolated systolic hypertensive group ($p = 0.05$). This is similar to a previous study that found that hypertension was positively associated with hearing loss. To be exact, results of audiometric examinations showed that the hypertensive group had a higher hearing capacity (23.4 ± 8.67 dB) in comparison with the non-hypertensive group (18.3 ± 6.02 dB), and the longer a person had had hypertension, the worse was their hearing ability [28]. Another study using audiometry also supported that a worse hearing level was found in hypertensive participants [29,30]. Emerging evidence proved that there was a gradually increasing level of a pure tone average (PTA) threshold and hearing impairment percentages at every frequency with an increase in the systolic standard deviation ($p < 0.05$) [31]. In 2019, Umesawa et al. tried to explore the mechanism behind the relationship between hearing impairment and hypertension. It was proven that bilateral hearing impairment was clearly caused by hypertension due to microvessel injury. Furthermore, they presumed that hypertension might damage both the inner ear organ and primary auditory cortex [32]. Additionally, a slightly increased risk of hearing impairment had a relationship with a history of hypertension [33].

Supporting our finding that hearing loss was associated with both age and hypertension, there is also a study that indicated that hypertension was related to age ($p < 0.001$) [34]. In addition, several lines of evidence showed that aging was positively associated with ISH, and ISH commonly occurred in young adults and the elderly [14,35,36]. We tried to make connections between those findings and other predictors. Although we observed that self-reported hypertension and having a general check-up were crucial predictors for avoiding hearing problems in adults aged 26~35 years, we did not find any previous study that supported those findings. Our findings in this study might be the first description of hearing problems being related to age and hypertension.

An increase in systolic blood pressure in early adults (26~35 years old) may be important, as it might increase the risk of hearing disturbances. So, we would encourage adults aged 26~35 years to have regular blood pressure check-ups and have early intervention if they have an elevated SBP in order to prevent hearing loss conditions. Moreover, this study emphasized the relationship between hearing problems and hypertension, and hence, this could be useful for future studies related to hypertension, especially in Indonesian populations.

Apart from the subjectivity of self-reported hearing loss and self-reported hypertension, only a few indicators related to hearing disturbances were available in this study. This survey also did not have noise exposure information. In addition, there was a discrepancy between self-reported hypertension with blood pressure measurement results, and some of the blood pressure measurements were non-responded cases. Another limitation was the respondents' volunteer effect, which might have been a factor that could have affected the results. We explored every variable which we thought to be useful in this study; however, these limitations were considerable since the survey mainly explored social aspects.

5. Conclusions

There was a predictive value of self-reported hypertension (awareness) and having a general check-up against hearing problems in early adults. Thus, regularly monitoring the blood pressure can be suggested for this age group. Future studies are needed to investigate the mechanism of these findings.

Supplementary Materials: The following supporting information can be downloaded at: https://www.mdpi.com/article/10.3390/ijerph19159222/s1, Table S1: Univariate logistic regression of hearing problem and demographic data based on gender; Table S2: Multivariate logistic regression analysis of hearing problem and demographic data based on gender.

Author Contributions: Conceptualization, M.F. and C.-H.B.; methodology, M.F. and C.-H.B.; software, M.F.; validation, C.-H.B.; formal analysis, M.F. and C.-H.B.; investigation, M.F. and C.-H.B.; resources, M.F. and C.-H.B.; data curation, M.F. and C.-H.B.; writing—original draft preparation, M.F. and C.-H.B.; writing—review and editing, C.-H.B.; visualization, M.F. and C.-H.B.; supervision, C.-H.B.; project administration, C.-H.B.; funding acquisition, C.-H.B. All authors have read and agreed to the published version of the manuscript.

Funding: This study was funded by the Ministry of Science and Technology, Taiwan, in the form of a grant awarded to CHB (reference number: MOST 107-2314-B-038-072-MY3 and MOST 110-2314-B038-056-MY3).

Institutional Review Board Statement: The IFLS survey had been authorized by RAND's ethics review boards as well as Universitas Gadjah Mada's ethics review boards in Indonesia.

Informed Consent Statement: Informed consent was obtained from all subjects involved prior to data collection.

Data Availability Statement: This research was conducted by using IFLS 5th waves provided by RAND (http://wwww.rand.org) and this database is open source. Last accessed on 1 May 2022.

Acknowledgments: The authors would like to thank the RAND Corporation for providing the survey data publicly and the participants in this survey. We are grateful to the Laboratory Animal Center at TMU for technical support in editorial and manuscript preparation.

Conflicts of Interest: The authors declare no conflict of interest.

References

1. *Global Costs of Unaddressed Hearing Loss and Cost-Effectiveness of Interventions: A WHO Report, 2017*; World Health Organization: Geneva, Switzerland, 2017.
2. *Addressing the Rising Prevalence of Hearing Loss*; World Health Organization: Geneva, Switzerland, 2018.
3. Miyata, J.; Umesawa, M.; Yoshioka, T.; Iso, H. Association between high systolic blood pressure and objective hearing impairment among Japanese adults: A facility-based retrospective cohort study. *Hypertens. Res.* **2022**, *45*, 155–161. [CrossRef] [PubMed]
4. Graydon, K.; Waterworth, C.; Miller, H.; Gunasekera, H. Global burden of hearing impairment and ear disease. *J. Laryngol. Otol.* **2019**, *133*, 18–25. [CrossRef] [PubMed]
5. Shukla, A.; Harper, M.; Pedersen, E.; Goman, A.; Suen, J.J.; Price, C.; Applebaum, J.; Hoyer, M.; Lin, F.R.; Reed, N.S. Hearing Loss, Loneliness, and Social Isolation: A Systematic Review. *Otolaryngol. Head Neck Surg.* **2020**, *162*, 622–633. [CrossRef] [PubMed]
6. Haile, L.M.; Kamenov, K.; Briant, P.S.; Orji, A.U.; Steinmetz, J.D.; Abdoli, A.; Rao, C.R. Hearing loss prevalence and years lived with disability, 1990-2019: Findings from the Global Burden of Disease Study 2019. *Lancet* **2021**, *397*, 996–1009. [CrossRef]
7. Mahboubi, H.; Lin, H.W.; Bhattacharyya, N. Prevalence, Characteristics, and Treatment Patterns of Hearing Difficulty in the United States. *JAMA Otolaryngol. Head Neck Surg.* **2018**, *144*, 65–70. [CrossRef]
8. Michels, T.C.; Duffy, M.T.; Rogers, D.J. Hearing Loss in Adults: Differential Diagnosis and Treatment. *Am. Fam. Physician* **2019**, *100*, 98–108.
9. Virani, S.S.; Alonso, A.; Aparicio, H.J.; Benjamin, E.J.; Bittencourt, M.S.; Callaway, C.W.; Carson, A.P.; Chamberlain, A.M.; Cheng, S.; Delling, F.N.; et al. Heart Disease and Stroke Statistics-2021 Update: A Report From the American Heart Association. *Circulation* **2021**, *143*, e254–e743. [CrossRef]
10. Mills, K.T.; Stefanescu, A.; He, J. The global epidemiology of hypertension. *Nat. Rev. Nephrol.* **2020**, *16*, 223–237. [CrossRef]
11. Roth, G.A.; Mensah, G.A.; Johnson, C.O.; Addolorato, G.; Ammirati, E.; Baddour, L.M.; Barengo, N.C.; Beaton, A.Z.; Benjamin, E.J.; Benziger, C.P.; et al. Global Burden of Cardiovascular Diseases and Risk Factors, 1990–2019: Update from the GBD 2019 Study. *J. Am. Coll. Cardiol.* **2020**, *76*, 2982–3021. [CrossRef]
12. Zhou, B.; Carrillo-Larco, R.M.; Danaei, G.; Riley, L.M.; Paciorek, C.J.; Stevens, G.A.; Breckenkamp, J. Worldwide trends in hypertension prevalence and progress in treatment and control from 1990 to 2019: A pooled analysis of 1201 population-representative studies with 104 million participants. *Lancet* **2021**, *398*, 957–980. [CrossRef]
13. Liu, J.; Bu, X.; Wei, L.; Wang, X.; Lai, L.; Dong, C.; Ma, A.; Wang, T. Global burden of cardiovascular diseases attributable to hypertension in young adults from 1990 to 2019. *J. Hypertens.* **2021**, *39*, 2488–2496. [CrossRef]
14. Tsai, T.Y.; Cheng, H.M.; Chuang, S.Y.; Chia, Y.C.; Soenarta, A.A.; Minh, H.V.; Siddique, S.; Turana, Y.; Tay, J.C.; Kario, K.; et al. Isolated systolic hypertension in Asia. *J. Clin. Hypertens.* **2021**, *23*, 467–474. [CrossRef]
15. Verulava, T.; Mikiashvili, G. Knowledge, awareness, attitude and medication compliance in patients with hypertension. *Arterial. Hypertens.* **2021**, *25*, 119–126. [CrossRef]
16. Tan, H.E.; Lan, N.S.R.; Knuiman, M.W.; Divitini, M.L.; Swanepoel, D.W.; Hunter, M.; Brennan-Jones, C.G.; Hung, J.; Eikelboom, R.H.; Santa Maria, P.L. Associations between cardiovascular disease and its risk factors with hearing loss-A cross-sectional analysis. *Clin. Otolaryngol.* **2018**, *43*, 172–181. [CrossRef]

17. Hara, K.; Okada, M.; Takagi, D.; Tanaka, K.; Senba, H.; Teraoka, M.; Yamada, H.; Matsuura, B.; Hato, N.; Miyake, Y. Association between hypertension, dyslipidemia, and diabetes and prevalence of hearing impairment in Japan. *Hypertens. Res.* **2020**, *43*, 963–968. [CrossRef]
18. Trune, D.R. Ion homeostasis in the ear: Mechanisms, maladies, and management. *Curr. Opin. Otolaryngol. Head Neck Surg.* **2010**, *18*, 413–419. [CrossRef]
19. Agarwal, S.; Mishra, A.; Jagade, M.; Kasbekar, V.; Nagle, S.K. Effects of hypertension on hearing. *Indian J. Otolaryngol. Head Neck Surg.* **2013**, *65*, 614–618. [CrossRef]
20. Lloyd-Jones, D.M.; Evans, J.C.; Larson, M.G.; O'Donnell, C.J.; Levy, D. Differential impact of systolic and diastolic blood pressure level on JNC-VI staging. Joint National Committee on Prevention, Detection, Evaluation, and Treatment of High Blood Pressure. *Hypertension* **1999**, *34*, 381–385. [CrossRef]
21. Chuang, S.Y.; Cheng, H.M.; Chou, P.; Chen, C.H. Prevalence of Isolated Systolic Hypertension and the Awareness, Treatment, and Control Rate of Hypertension in Kinmen. *Acta. Cardiol. Sin.* **2006**, *22*, 83–90.
22. Strauss, J.; Witoelar, F.; Sikoki, B. *The Fifth Wave of the Indonesia Family Life Survey (IFLS5): Overview and Field Report*; Rand: Santa Monica, CA, USA, 2016.
23. Whelton, P.K.; Carey, R.M.; Aronow, W.S.; Casey, D.E., Jr.; Collins, K.J.; Dennison Himmelfarb, C.; DePalma, S.M.; Gidding, S.; Jamerson, K.A.; Jones, D.W.; et al. 2017 ACC/AHA/AAPA/ABC/ACPM/AGS/APhA/ASH/ASPC/NMA/PCNA Guideline for the Prevention, Detection, Evaluation, and Management of High Blood Pressure in Adults: A Report of the American College of Cardiology/American Heart Association Task Force on Clinical Practice Guidelines. *J. Am. Coll. Cardiol.* **2018**, *71*, e127–e248. [CrossRef]
24. Williams, B.; Mancia, G.; Spiering, W.; Agabiti Rosei, E.; Azizi, M.; Burnier, M.; Clement, D.L.; Coca, A.; de Simone, G.; Dominiczak, A.; et al. 2018 ESC/ESH Guidelines for the management of arterial hypertension: The Task Force for the management of arterial hypertension of the European Society of Cardiology and the European Society of Hypertension. *J. Hypertens.* **2018**, *36*, 1953–2041. [CrossRef] [PubMed]
25. *World Report on Hearing*; World Health Organization: Geneva, Switzerland, 2021.
26. Hoffman, H.J.; Dobie, R.A.; Losonczy, K.G.; Themann, C.L.; Flamme, G.A. Declining Prevalence of Hearing Loss in US Adults Aged 20 to 69 Years. *JAMA Otolaryngol. Head Neck Surg.* **2017**, *143*, 274–285. [CrossRef]
27. Ramage-Morin, P.L.; Gilmour, H.; Banks, R.; Pineault, D.; Atrach, M. Hypertension associated with hearing health problems among Canadian adults aged 19 to 79 years. *Health Rep.* **2021**, *32*, 14–26. [CrossRef]
28. Nawaz, M.U.; Vinayak, S.; Rivera, E.; Elahi, K.; Tahir, H.; Ahuja, V.; Jogezai, S.; Maher, W.; Naz, S. Association Between Hypertension and Hearing Loss. *Cureus* **2021**, *13*, e18025. [CrossRef]
29. Yikawe, S.S.; Uguru, S.U.; Solomon, J.H.; Adamu, A.M.; Damtong, F.; Osisi, K.; Adeyeye, F.M. Hearing loss among hypertensive patients. *Egypt. J. Otolaryngol.* **2019**, *35*, 307–312. [CrossRef]
30. Samelli, A.G.; Santos, I.S.; Padilha, F.; Gomes, R.F.; Moreira, R.R.; Rabelo, C.M.; Matas, C.G.; Bensenor, I.M.; Lotufo, P.A. Hearing loss, tinnitus, and hypertension: Analysis of the baseline data from the Brazilian Longitudinal Study of Adult Health (ELSA-Brasil). *Clinics* **2021**, *76*, e2370. [CrossRef]
31. Bao, M.; Song, Y.; Cai, J.; Wu, S.; Yang, X. Blood Pressure Variability Is Associated with Hearing and Hearing Loss: A Population-Based Study in Males. *Int. J. Hypertens.* **2019**, *2019*, 9891025. [CrossRef]
32. Umesawa, M.; Sairenchi, T.; Haruyama, Y.; Nagao, M.; Kobashi, G. Association between hypertension and hearing impairment in health check-ups among Japanese workers: A cross-sectional study. *BMJ Open* **2019**, *9*, e028392. [CrossRef] [PubMed]
33. Lin, B.M.; Curhan, S.G.; Wang, M.; Eavey, R.; Stankovic, K.M.; Curhan, G.C. Hypertension, Diuretic Use, and Risk of Hearing Loss. *Am. J. Med.* **2016**, *129*, 416–422. [CrossRef]
34. Peltzer, K.; Pengpid, S. The Prevalence and Social Determinants of Hypertension among Adults in Indonesia: A Cross-Sectional Population-Based National Survey. *Int. J. Hypertens.* **2018**, *2018*, 5610725. [CrossRef]
35. Scott, H.; Barton, M.J.; Johnston, A.N.B. Isolated systolic hypertension in young males: A scoping review. *Clin. Hypertens.* **2021**, *27*, 12. [CrossRef] [PubMed]
36. Xie, K.; Gao, X.; Bao, L.; Shan, Y.; Shi, H.; Li, Y. The different risk factors for isolated diastolic hypertension and isolated systolic hypertension: A national survey. *BMC Public Health* **2021**, *21*, 1672. [CrossRef] [PubMed]

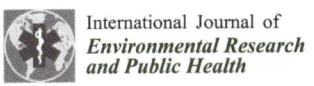

Article

Swallowing Outcomes in Open Partial Horizontal Laryngectomy Type I and Endoscopic Supraglottic Laryngectomy: A Comparative Study

Carmelo Saraniti [1], Francesco Ciodaro [2], Cosimo Galletti [2], Salvatore Gallina [1] and Barbara Verro [1,*]

[1] Division of Otorhinolaryngology, Department of Biomedicine, Neuroscience and Advanced Diagnostic, University of Palermo, 90127 Palermo, Italy; carmelo.saraniti@unipa.it (C.S.); salvatore.gallina@unipa.it (S.G.)
[2] Division of Otorhinolaryngology, Department of Adult and Development Age Human Pathology "Gaetano Barresi", University of Messina, 98125 Messina, Italy; dottfciodaro@alice.it (F.C.); cosimogalletti92@gmail.com (C.G.)
* Correspondence: verrobarbara@gmail.com; Tel.: +39-327-1722-000

Abstract: Background: Effective swallowing represents the main challenge in supraglottic laryngectomy. This study aimed to assess swallowing outcome comparing endoscopic supraglottic laryngectomy (ESL) and open partial horizontal laryngectomy type I (OPHL I). **Methods:** A retrospective study was carried out on 20 patients that underwent supraglottic laryngectomy from 2015 to 2021: 10 underwent ESL (group A) and 10 underwent OPHL I (Group B). Patients underwent fiberoptic endoscopic evaluation of swallowing (FEES) 3 months and 12 months after surgery and videofluoroscopy swallowing studies (VFSS) 12 months after surgery. A Swallowing Outcome After Laryngectomy (SOAL) questionnaire was administered to patients to assess their life quality. **Results:** A naso-gastric tube was placed in two patients of Group A and in all patients of Group B. Tracheostomy was performed in two patients of Group A and in all patients in Group B and it has been closed in 100% of them. According to Donzelli's scale, FEES and VFSS showed better results in Group A at 3 months, while at 12 months they did not show statistically significant differences between ESL and OPHL I in terms of laryngeal penetration and aspiration. The SOAL questionnaire showed satisfactory life quality. **Conclusion:** Swallowing evaluation by FEES and VFSS did not demonstrate statistically significant differences at 12 months post-op between two surgeries, although ESL showed less cases of laryngeal penetration and aspiration at 3 months post-op. Anyway, good results of any surgery depend on careful patient selection and the surgeon's experience.

Keywords: supraglottic laryngectomy; swallowing; partial laryngectomy; head and neck; surgical oncology

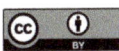

1. Introduction

Squamous cell carcinoma (Scc) represents about 98% of laryngeal cancers. In particular, the supraglottis is the second most common laryngeal region affected by carcinoma (about 30%) [1].

In this laryngeal region, the tumor remains usually asymptomatic in the early stage; few and non-specific symptoms, as dysphagia or reflex otalgia, occur in advanced stage. Due to this attitude, diagnosis is often late and so prognosis of supraglottic cancer is poor [2]. Currently, T1-T2 supraglottic tumors can be treated by different strategies: radiotherapy (RT), transoral laser microsurgery (TLM) or open supraglottic laryngectomy (OPHL type I) [3,4]. The main goals of the treatment are: oncological radicality and organ and function preservation, in terms of swallowing, speaking and breathing. Recent studies found that TLM ensures organ preservation with poor impairment of laryngeal functions compared to other therapeutic approaches [3,5,6]. However, a careful pre-operative assessment of the patient is crucial for detection of the best therapeutic choice; in fact, it depends on the patient's age, on his comorbidity and on tumor extension [7]. In particular, in 2009, the European Laryngological Society (ELS) proposed a classification of endoscopic supraglottic laryngectomy (ESL) [8] describing four types of TLM depending on tumor extension: limited excision of the small tumor (type I); medial supraglottic laryngectomy with partial resection of the pre-epiglottic space above (type IIa) or below (type IIb) hyoid bone; medial supraglottic laryngectomy with resection of the pre-epiglottic space for tumors extending to the petiole of epiglottis (type IIIa) or to ventricular folds (type IIIb); lateral supraglottic laryngectomy including the free edge of the epiglottis, threefolds' region and ventricular folds (type Iva) or extending to the arytenoid (type IVb). This kind of surgery is indicated for T1-T2 tumors, without impairment of cordal function. On the other side, in 2014, ELS stated the classification of OPHL [9], defining three types: supraglottic (type I), supracricoid (type II) and supratracheal (type III) laryngectomy, depending on inferior limited resection. Moreover, in this case, the resection could extend to one arytenoid (ARY), base of tongue (BOT), one piriform sinus (PIR) or one crico-arytenoid unit (CAU).

The main challenge in supraglottic laryngectomy (ESL or open) is represented by valid and effective swallowing since the resected anatomical structures play an important role in airway protection during swallowing. So, in this study, we compared the two surgical techniques in order to define limits and advantages in terms of swallowing.

2. Materials and Methods

A retrospective study was carried out on patients that underwent supraglottic laryngectomy (ESL or open) in our ENT Clinics from January 2010 to December 2020. Informed consent to participate in the study was obtained from the patients and the study was approved by the ethics committee of our University Hospital. Inclusion criteria were: males and females, aged between 18 and 65 years old, with supraglottic Scc, T1-T2 according to criteria of the American Joint Committee on Cancer (AJCC), eligible for surgery (ESL type III–IV or OPHL type I), negative resection margin status and pN0. Concerning resection margin status, we assumed the cut-off of 1 mm as margin-tumor distance to distinguish between close and negative margins [10]. Exclusion criteria were: pre-operative and/or post-operative chemoradiation therapy (ChRT), previous other head and neck surgeries (except for the diagnostic biopsy), neurologic diseases, contraindication to fiberoptic endoscopic evaluation of swallowing (FEES) [11] and/or videofluoroscopy swallowing study (VFSS) [12] and previous oropharyngeal dysphagia. These strict criteria allowed to select patients of the two groups that were similar in all respects (age, sex, without pre-op and/or post-op ChRT and without other causes of impaired swallowing regardless of ELS or OPHL I). Doing so, we tried to avoid bias in the results due to the significant differences of the two groups that would have made the comparison of the two surgeries impossible.

2.1. Study Protocol

Recruited patients were divided into two groups depending on surgery: ESL (group A) and OPHL type I (group B). At a post-operative time, patients performed supraglottic swallowing exercises.

Patients underwent FEES twice: three months and one year after surgery. FEES was performed by the same dysphagia expert otorhinolaryngologist (CS). During the exam, we first tested laryngeal perception by the touch method [13]: we touch the laryngeal mucosa with the tip of the flexible laryngoscope in order to elicit a cough, gag or laryngeal adductor reflex and to evaluate any damage on the internal branch of superior laryngeal nerve. Recurrent laryngeal nerve function was assessed by phonatory exercises, breath holding and coughing. Then, the patient, in a sitting position, had to swallow two different food textures: liquid (water with green food dye) and thickened liquid (yogurt). The tip of a flexible endoscope was positioned beyond the soft palate and the pharyngeal phase of swallowing was studied recording videos and images for further analysis. In particular, according to the Donzelli secretion severity scale, the following parameters were assessed: pharyngeal residue, laryngeal penetration and tracheal aspiration. It is a three-point scale: level 1, functional, if there is pharyngeal residue without penetration or aspiration; level 2, severe, if secretion reaches laryngeal vestibule; level 3, profound, in case of tracheal aspiration [14,15].

One year after surgery, patients underwent VFSS: during the exam, patients had to swallow different textures of liquid (barium solution diluted with different volume of water) and antero-posterior and lateral fluoroscopic video images were recorded at a speed of 15 frames per second. These images were studied by the same radiologist with great experience in VFSS who investigated the same parameters—pharyngeal residue, laryngeal penetration, tracheal aspiration—according to Donzelli's scoring scale.

One year after surgery, each patient was administered the Italian version of Swallowing Outcome After Laryngectomy (SOAL) questionnaire to assess their quality of life related to dysphagia [15,16]. This self-administered questionnaire consists of 17 items with multiple-choice answers: no; a little; a lot. Moreover, if patients answered "a little" or "a lot", then they had to indicate if this bothered them.

Moreover, in the assessment of the functional outcome, duration of naso-gastric feeding, need of Percutaneous Endoscopic Gastrostomy (PEG) and/or persistence of tracheostomy had also been assessed.

2.2. Data Analysis

Demographic and medical data, type and subtype of surgery, tumor staging and grade of differentiation and resection margin status about recruited patients were collected in a data spreadsheet using the Microsoft Excel version 16.47.1. Results were reported as numbers, percentages of the total and/or mean ± standard deviation (SD). Chi-square tests with Yates correction were performed to compare the two groups (A and B) using MedCalc Statistical Software (MedCalc Software Ltd., Ostend, Belgium).

3. Results

The study included 20 patients: 4 females and 16 males, aged between 42 and 65 years old (mean age was 59.5 ± 4.91). Out of 20 patients, 10 underwent ESL (group A) and 10 underwent OPHL type I (Group B). In particular, Group A included: six type IIIa, two type IIIb and two type IVa. No endoscopic supraglottic laryngectomy type IVb was performed. Included patients had pT1-T2N0 supraglottic tumors with close or negative resection margins, so they did not need adjuvant therapy. Patients with close resection margins received a closer follow-up than patients with negative margins. Data are reported in Table 1.

Table 1. Patients' characteristics.

Characteristics	N (%)
Sex	
Male	16 (80)
Group A	10
Group B	6
Female	4 (20)
Group A	0
Group B	4
Age (years)	
Mean (± SD)	59.5 ± 4.91
Group A	60.8 ± 3.25
Group B	58.3 ± 5.88
Range	42–65
Group A	56–65
Group B	60–65

Table 1. *Cont.*

Characteristics	N (%)	
ESL (Group A)		
Type IIIa	6 (60)	
Type IIIb	2 (20)	
Type IVa	2 (20)	
Type IVb	0 (0)	
OPHL I (Group B)	10	
Superior laryngeal nerve integrity (touch method)		
Group A	10	
Group B	10	
Duration of naso-gastric feeding (days)		
Group A		
Patient #2	2	
Patients #5	4	
Group B	14	
PEG		
Group A	0	
Group B	0	
Need of tracheostomy		
Group A	2	
Group B	10	
Permanent tracheostomy		
Group A	0	
Group B	0	
Hospitalization time (days)		
Mean ± SD		
Group A	12.5 ± 6.15	
Group B	27.5 ± 5.83	
Range		
Group A	6–26	
Group B	18–45	
Post-op complications	Group A	Group B
Bleeding	0	2 (20)
Prelaryngeal abscess	0	1 (10)
Edema	2 (20)	0
Chondritis	0	0
Aspiration pneumonia	0	0
Laryngeal stenosis	0	0
pT	Group A	Group B
T1	7	5
T2	3	5
Grade of differentiation	Group A	Group B
G1	3	0
G2	4	6
G3	3	4
Resection margin status	Group A	Group B
Close (<1 mm)	4	3
Negative (>1 mm)	6	7
Total	20 (100)	

SD: standard deviation; ESL: endoscopic supraglottic laryngectomy; OPHL: open partial horizontal laryngectomy; PEG: Percutaneous Endoscopic Gastrostomy; pT: pathological stage of tumor; G1: low grade or well-differentiated tumor; G2: moderate grade or moderately differentiated tumor; G3: high grade or poorly differentiated tumor.

3.1. FEES and VFSS

Three months after surgery, the touch method by endoscopy did not show impaired laryngeal perception in either group. Analyzing the FEES exam, Group A showed better results than Group B. In the former group, nobody had pharyngeal residue and/or tracheal aspiration. Only six patients (60%) had laryngeal penetration swallowing water (level 2 according to Donzelli's score): two patients underwent ESL type IIIa, two patients ESL type IIIb and two patients ESL type IVa. As regards Group B, we found two patients with pharyngeal residue swallowing yogurt (level 1) and two patients with water in the laryngeal vestibule (level 2) and six patients with tracheal aspiration (level 3), according to Donzelli's scale. At 12 months after surgery, eight patients (80%) of Group A showed a worsening swallowing, while on the contrary four patients (40%) of Group B had an improvement in swallowing and the other six (60%) showed no changes. VFSS, performed twelve months after surgery, showed the same results of FEES as regards Group A; instead, in Group B, we found the following results: level 1 in two patients, level 2 in two patients and level 3 in six patients. So, for Group B, FEES and VFSS findings were not perfectly overlapping, with more episodes of tracheal aspiration during VFSS. FEES and VFSS results are reported in Table 2.

Table 2. FEES and VFSS results.

Group	Sex	Age	Surgery	FEES		VFSS
				3 Months *	12 Months *	12 Months *
Group A			ELS			
#1	M	58	IIIa	No dysphagia	Level 1	Level 1
#2	M	56	IVa	Level 2	Level 2	Level 2
#3	M	65	IIIb	Level 2	Level 3	Level 3
#4	M	63	IIIa	No dysphagia	Level 2	Level 2
#5	M	65	IIIa	Level 2	Level 3	Level 3
#6	M	58	IIIb	Level 2	Level 3	Level 3
#7	M	57	IIIa	No dysphagia	Level 1	Level 1
#8	M	64	IIIa	No dysphagia	Level 2	Level 2
#9	M	60	IVa	Level 2	Level 2	Level 2
#10	M	62	IIIa	Level 2	Level 3	Level 3
Group B						
#11	M	60	OPHL I	Level 3	Level 2	Level 3
#12	F	42	OPHL I	Level 2	Level 2	Level 2
#13	F	60	OPHL I	Level 1	Level 1	Level 1
#14	M	62	OPHL I	Level 3	Level 2	Level 3
#15	M	65	OPHL I	Level 3	Level 3	Level 3
#16	M	56	OPHL I	Level 2	Level 2	Level 2
#17	F	60	OPHL I	Level 1	Level 1	Level 1
#18	M	59	OPHL I	Level 3	Level 2	Level 3
#19	F	58	OPHL I	Level 3	Level 2	Level 3
#20	M	61	OPHL I	Level 3	Level 3	Level 3

* after surgery.

Comparing the *food in laryngeal vestibule* parameter between the two groups based on the FEES results, we did not find statistically significant relationships between this parameter and the type of surgery (ESL vs. OPHL I): the chi-square statistic with Yates correction was 0.952 (p-value 0.32) and 0.312 (p-value 0.57), respectively, 3 months and 12 months after surgery.

3.2. Post-Operative Outcome

A naso-gastric tube was placed only in two patients of Group A (#2 and #5) and in all patients of Group B and removed on the 14th post-operative day in Group B, on the 4th post-operative day in patient #2 and on the 2nd post-operative day in patient #5. No patients needed a PEG. A tracheostomy was performed in all patients in Group B and it has been closed in 100% of them. As for Group A, a covering tracheostomy was performed in two patients (#2 and #5) during ESL: one patient underwent ESL type IIIa and one patient underwent ESL type IVa. In these two cases, covering tracheostomy was performed due to a swelling airway after surgery. However, the tracheostomy was closed a few weeks after surgery. It should be noted that, during the first FEES, swallowing worsened in Group A and was found in these two tracheostomized patients.

Hospitalization lasted less in case of ESL (12.5 ± 6.15). Post-operative bleeding occurred in only two patients, both of Group B. No other complications have been detected.

3.3. SOAL Questionnaire

Overall, the SOAL questionnaire showed a good and satisfactory quality of life without an impairment due to swallowing problems (Table 3). In particular, patients (6/20) reported problems swallowing thin liquids (item #2) and dry solid food (item #5). Of these six patients, four belonged to the Group B. Moreover, few patients answered that they took longer to eat a meal (item #12) and reduced the size of their meal (item #14). In conclusion, these swallowing problems did not affect their quality of life.

Table 3. Swallowing outcome after laryngectomy (SOAL) questionnaire [16] (one year after surgery).

	Items	Not	A Little	A Lot	If You Answered "a Little" or "a Lot", Please Indicate if This Bothers You
1	In your opinion, do you have a swallowing problem now?	16	4	0	0
2	Do you have a problem swallowing thin liquids (water ...)?	14	6	0	0
3	Do you have a problem swallowing thick liquids (soup ...)?	20	0	0	-
4	Do you have a problem swallowing soft/mashed foods?	20	0	0	-
5	Do you have a problem swallowing dry solid food (bread ...)?	14	6	0	0
6	Do liquids stick in your throat when you swallow?	18	2	0	0
7	Does food stick in your throat when you swallow?	16	4	0	0
8	Does food or liquid come back up into your mouth or nose when you eat or drink?	20	0	0	-
9	Do you need to swallow liquid to help the food go down?	18	2	0	0
10	Do you need to swallow many times on each mouthful to help the food or drink go down?	18	20	0	0
11	Do you avoid certain food because you cannot swallow them?	16	4	0	0
12	Does it take longer to eat a meal?	14	6	0	0
13	Has your enjoyment of food reduced?	20	0	0	-
14	Has the size of your meal reduced?	12	8	0	0
15	Has your appetite reduced because you cannot taste or smell food normally?	20	0	0	-
16	Has your eating been more difficult due to dry mouth?	16	4	0	0
17	Do you feel self-conscious eating with other people?	18	2	0	0

Value reported as numbers.

4. Discussion

There are several treatments for T1-T2 supraglottic cancer: radiotherapy, TLM, transoral robotic surgery (TORS) and open partial horizontal laryngectomy (OPHL). Each therapeutic approach has proven effective in terms of survival rates and local control: in particular, five-year local control rates range from about 75% to 100% and from about 60% to 80%, respectively, for T1 and for T2 supraglottic cancers regardless of the therapy [17]. As recommended in 2018 by the American Society of Clinical Oncology (ASCO), the best treatment for limited-stage (T1-T2) laryngeal cancer should have three goals: curing the cancer, preserving organ functions, and ensuring satisfactory quality of life [18]. The ASCO also stated that this optimal treatment can be achieved through a full and multidisciplinary evaluation of patients in terms of cancer staging and tumor characteristics (tumor size, local-regional extension), health and socioeconomic, psychosocial state and choice of patient and logistic issue [8,18–20]. Moreover, the treatment choice depends on surgeon expertise and availability of rehabilitative experts. However, the main and final issue is to avoid combined-modality therapy (surgery plus RT) because it can impair functional outcomes. According to these international guidelines and recommendations, we performed ELS or OPHL type I, keeping in mind that, also in experienced hands, the therapeutic choice depends mainly on laryngeal exposure to achieve tumor-free margins [8,18]. The open horizontal supraglottic laryngectomy was first described by Alonso in 1947 [21]. About 30 years later, in 1972, Strong et al. described the endoscopic supraglottic laryngectomy for the first time [22]. Moreover, a key problem related to both surgical and non-surgical treatments is impairment of swallowing. So, it represents the main challenge of surgical treatment for supraglottic tumors. For this reason, we decided to assess swallowing impairment and improvement in two group of patients: Group A underwent ESL and Group B underwent OPHL type I. We analyzed their swallowing residual function by FEES and VFSS exams, performed 3 months and 12 months after surgery. We found satisfying results in both groups, better in ESL patients. Moreover, we found no statistically significant different results at 12 months and an improvement in Group B. So, our study demonstrates that swallowing recovery is slower but similar in the case of OPHL than ESL. This finding is consistent with literature [7] and it could be explained by the reduced invasiveness of TLM, without sutures, strap muscles and thyroid cartilage involved and neither routine tracheostomy. Indeed, in our sample, ESL patients, who needed a covering tracheostomy, had worse swallowing at the beginning, probably due to the tracheostomy itself. The good results in both groups could also be explained by the preservation of the superior laryngeal nerve achieved in all patients.

Contrary to Peretti et al.'s study [23], we did not find any statistically significant differences between two therapeutic approaches for FEES. Further, in our study, tracheal aspiration was more frequent in VFSS than in FEES. Actually, although VFSS does not provide anatomic and function details, it can detect minor aspiration events. For this reason, the two exams are necessary and complementary for a comprehensive assessment of swallowing. In this regard, a study reported that, in patients undergoing supraglottic laryngectomy, tracheal aspiration events were more frequent post-swallowing rather than intra- or pre-swallowing [24].

In our study, in addition to the objective analysis of swallowing (FEES and VFSS), we also performed a subjective evaluation of the quality of life related to swallowing. The one-year SOAL questionnaire—created specifically for laryngectomized patients—showed good and satisfactory quality of life in both groups, although with minor swallowing impairment that did not affect their lives anyway. Similar results found Peretti et al. administering the M.D. Anderson Dysphagia Inventory (MDADI) questionnaire [23,25]. However, we should point out that results of the questionnaire between both groups cannot be compared because they are two different surgical techniques and patients' lives facing two different swallowing difficulties and problems.

In our study, we evaluated the duration of naso-gastric feeding. In several studies, the naso-gastric tube was placed in almost all ESL patients [7,24,26]. On the contrary, we placed a naso-gastric tube only in two ESL patients and it was removed early. Additionally, a tracheostomy was performed in just two ESL patients due to swelling airways. However, we closed the tracheostomy on both of the patients. No patient, in either group, needed a permanent tracheostomy. This result is quite consistent with current literature [7,23]. In our case series, hospitalization lasted on average 12.5 ± 6.15 days and 27.5 ± 5.83 days for Group A and B, respectively: as expected and reported in literature [7,23], ESL has a faster recovery with a lower mean hospitalization than OPHL. Moreover, like all surgeries, supraglottic laryngectomies also run the risk of complications: post-surgical bleeding, neck abscess, chondritis of thyroid cartilage, aspiration pneumonia, laryngeal stenosis and pharyngocutaneous fistulas [7]. Aspiration pneumonia, need of tracheostomy and bleeding represent the main complications reported in literature. In our case series, we encountered only two cases of post-operative bleeding, both in Group B, and as reported above, two cases of temporary tracheostomy due to post-operative laryngeal swelling in Group A. No other complications have been encountered. Current literature did not demonstrate any statistically significant difference in aspiration pneumonia rate between these two types of surgeries [7,26].

Anyway, our study had a main limit: the small sample size. So, our results need to be confirmed by other studies. Indeed, to achieve the most homogeneous sample possible we included only patients who underwent ESL type III or IV with a wider resection, comparable to OPHL. Moreover, we have excluded patients over the age of 65 in order to avoid bias related to presbyphagia. For the same reason, we also excluded patients who underwent pre-operative and/or post-operative ChRT because it can impair swallowing. FEES and VFSS were always performed by the same specialists in order to avoid bias related to different performance of the examination and interpretation of the results.

5. Conclusions

Supraglottic carcinoma surgery, both endoscopic and transcervical, was born with the main aim of reaching oncological radicality with safe resection margins and, at the same time, the preservation of laryngeal functions. From our analysis of the swallowing outcome, endoscopic surgery resulted better at 3 months post-op, but 12 months swallowing results did not show statistically significant differences in terms of laryngeal penetration and aspiration between the two surgeries. Anyway, good and appreciated oncological and functional results of each surgical technique depend on two main factors: careful patient selection and the surgeon's experience.

6. Highlights

- The main goals of supraglottic carcinoma surgery are oncological radicality and organ and function preservation;
- Supraglottic carcinoma surgery can be endoscopic (ESL) or transcervical (OPHL I);
- Swallowing results are better in ESL at 3 months post-op, but at 12 months post-op the two surgeries do not show statistically significant different results;
- Results of surgical techniques depend on careful patient selection and the surgeon's experience.

Author Contributions: Methodology, C.S., S.G.; validation, C.S., F.C.; formal analysis F.C.; investigation, B.V., C.G.; resources, B.V.; data curation, B.V., C.G.; writing—original draft preparation, B.V., C.G.; writing—review and editing, C.S., F.C.; supervision, C.S., S.G. All authors have read and agreed to the published version of the manuscript.

Funding: This research received no external funding.

Institutional Review Board Statement: The study was conducted in accordance with the Declaration of Helsinki and approved by the Ethics Committee Palermo 1 of University Hospital Paolo Giaccone, Palermo (protocol code 04/2021 and 28 April 2021).

Informed Consent Statement: Informed consent was obtained from all subjects involved in the study.

Data Availability Statement: Not applicable.

Conflicts of Interest: The authors declare no conflict of interest.

References

1. Nocini, R.; Molteni, G.; Mattiuzzi, C.; Lippi, G. Updates on larynx cancer epidemiology. *Chin. J. Cancer Res.* **2020**, *32*, 18–25. [CrossRef] [PubMed]
2. Patel, T.D.; Echanique, K.A.; Yip, C.; Hsueh, W.D.; Baredes, S.; Park, R.C.W.; Eloy, J.A. Supraglottic Squamous Cell Carcinoma: A Population-Based Study of 22,675 Cases. *Laryngoscope* **2018**, *129*, 1822–1827. [CrossRef] [PubMed]
3. Ambrosch, P.; Gonzalez-Donate, M.; Fazel, A.; Schmalz, C.; Hedderich, J. Transoral Laser Microsurgery for Supraglottic Cancer. *Front. Oncol.* **2018**, *8*, 158. [CrossRef] [PubMed]

4. Verro, B.; Greco, G.; Chianetta, E.; Saraniti, C. Management of Early Glottic Cancer Treated by CO_2 Laser According to Surgical-Margin Status: A Systematic Review of the Literature. *Int. Arch. Otorhinolaryngol.* **2020**, *25*, e301–e308. [CrossRef] [PubMed]
5. Swanson, M.; Low, G.; Sinha, U.K.; Kokot, N. Transoral surgery vs intensity-modulated radiotherapy for early supraglottic cancer: A systematic review. *Curr. Opin. Otolaryngol. Head Neck Surg.* **2017**, *25*, 133–141. [CrossRef] [PubMed]
6. Saraniti, C.; Montana, F.; Chianetta, E.; Greco, G.; Verro, B. Impact of resection margin status and revision transoral laser microsurgery in early glottic cancer: Analysis of organ preservation and local disease control on a cohort of 153 patients. *Braz. J. Otorhinolaryngol.* **2020**, *in press*. [CrossRef] [PubMed]
7. Estomba, C.C.; Reinoso, F.B.; Lorenzo, A.L.; Conde, J.F.; Nores, J.A.; Hidalgo, C.S. Functional outcomes of supraglottic squamous cell carcinoma treated by transoral laser microsurgery compared with horizontal supraglottic laryngectomy in patients younger and older than 65 years. Risultati funzionali in pazienti over e under 65 affetti da carcinoma squamocellulare sopraglottico trattati con chirurgia laser trans-orale o tradizionale laringectomia orizzontale sopraglottica. *Acta Otorhinolaryngol. Ital.* **2016**, *36*, 450–458. [CrossRef]
8. Remacle, M.; Hantzakos, A.; Eckel, H.; Evrard, A.-S.; Bradley, P.J.; Chevalier, D.; Djukic, V.; de Vincentiis, M.; Friedrich, G.; Olofsson, J.; et al. Endoscopic supraglottic laryngectomy: A proposal for a classification by the working committee on nomenclature, European Laryngological Society. *Eur. Arch. Otorhinolaryngol.* **2009**, *266*, 993–998. [CrossRef]
9. Succo, G.; Peretti, G.; Piazza, C.; Remacle, M.; Eckel, H.E.; Chevalier, D.; Simo, R.; Hantzakos, A.G.; Rizzotto, G.; Lucioni, M.; et al. Open partial horizontal laryngectomies: A proposal for classification by the working committee on nomenclature of the European Laryngological Society. *Eur. Arch. Otorhinolaryngol.* **2014**, *271*, 2489–2496. [CrossRef]
10. Osuch-Wójcikiewicz, E.; Rzepakowska, A.; Sobol, M.; Bruzgielewicz, A.; Niemczyk, K. Oncological outcomes of CO_2 laser cordectomies for glottic squamous cell carcinoma with respect to anterior commissure involvement and margin status. *Lasers Surg. Med.* **2019**, *51*, 874–881. [CrossRef]
11. Langmore, S.E. History of Fiberoptic Endoscopic Evaluation of Swallowing for Evaluation and Management of Pharyngeal Dysphagia: Changes over the Years. *Dysphagia* **2017**, *32*, 27–38. [CrossRef] [PubMed]
12. Kim, S.Y.; Kim, T.U.; Hyun, J.K.; Lee, S.J. Differences in Videofluoroscopic Swallowing Study (VFSS) Findings according to the Vascular Territory Involved in Stroke. *Dysphagia* **2014**, *29*, 444–449. [CrossRef] [PubMed]
13. Kaneoka, A.; Pisegna, J.; Inokuchi, H.; Ueha, R.; Goto, T.; Nito, T.; Stepp, C.E.; LaValley, M.; Haga, N.; Langmore, S.E. Relationship Between Laryngeal Sensory Deficits, Aspiration, and Pneumonia in Patients with Dysphagia. *Dysphagia* **2017**, *33*, 192–199. [CrossRef] [PubMed]
14. Donzelli, J.; Wesling, M.; Brady, S.; Craney, M. Predictive Value of Accumulated Oropharyngeal Secretions for Aspiration during Video Nasal Endoscopic Evaluation of the Swallow. *Ann. Otol. Rhinol. Laryngol.* **2003**, *112*, 469–475. [CrossRef]
15. Saraniti, C.; Speciale, R.; Santangelo, M.; Massaro, N.; Maniaci, A.; Gallina, S.; Serra, A.; Cocuzza, S. Functional outcomes after supracricoid modified partial laryngectomy. *J. Biol. Regul. Homeost. Agents* **2019**, *33*, 1903–1907. [CrossRef]
16. Govender, R.; Lee, M.; Davies, T.; Twinn, C.; Katsoulis, K.; Payten, C.L.; Stephens, R.; Drinnan, M. Development and preliminary validation of a patient-reported outcome measure for swallowing after total laryngectomy (SOAL questionnaire). *Clin. Otolaryngol.* **2012**, *37*, 452–459. [CrossRef]
17. Jones, T.M.; De, M.; Foran, B.; Harrington, K.; Mortimore, S. Laryngeal cancer: United Kingdom National Multidisciplinary guidelines. *J. Laryngol. Otol.* **2016**, *130*, S75–S82. [CrossRef]
18. Forastiere, A.A.; Ismaila, N.; Lewin, J.; Nathan, C.A.; Adelstein, D.J.; Eisbruch, A.; Fass, G.; Fisher, S.G.; Laurie, S.A.; Le, Q.-T.; et al. Use of Larynx-Preservation Strategies in the Treatment of Laryngeal Cancer: American Society of Clinical Oncology Clinical Practice Guideline Update. *J. Clin. Oncol.* **2018**, *36*, 1143–1169. [CrossRef]
19. Saraniti, C.; Verro, B.; Ciodaro, F.; Galletti, F. Oncological Outcomes of Primary vs. Salvage OPHL Type II: A Systematic Review. *Int. J. Environ. Res. Public Health* **2022**, *19*, 1837. [CrossRef]
20. Sperry, S.M.; Rassekh, C.H.; Laccourreye, O.; Weinstein, G.S. Supracricoid Partial Laryngectomy for Primary and Recurrent Laryngeal Cancer. *JAMA Otolaryngol. Neck Surg.* **2013**, *139*, 1226. [CrossRef]
21. Alonso, J.M. Conservative surgery of cancer of the larynx. *Trans. Am. Acad. Ophthalmol. Otolaryngol.* **1947**, *51*, 633–642. [PubMed]
22. Strong, M.S.; Jako, G.J. Laser Surgery in the Larynx Early Clinical Experience with Continuous CO_2 Laser. *Ann. Otol. Rhinol. Laryngol.* **1972**, *81*, 791–798. [CrossRef] [PubMed]
23. Peretti, G.; Piazza, C.; Cattaneo, A.; De Benedetto, L.; Martin, E.; Nicolai, P. Comparison of Functional Outcomes after Endoscopic versus Open-Neck Supraglottic Laryngectomies. *Ann. Otol. Rhinol. Laryngol.* **2006**, *115*, 827–832. [CrossRef] [PubMed]
24. Prgomet, D.; Bumber, Z.; Bilić, M.; Svoren, E.; Katić, V.; Poje, G. Videofluoroscopy of the swallowing act after partial supraglottic laryngectomy by CO_2 laser. *Eur. Arch. Otorhinolaryngol.* **2002**, *259*, 399–403. [CrossRef] [PubMed]
25. Chen, A.Y.; Frankowski, R.; Bishop-Leone, J.; Hebert, T.; Leyk, S.; Lewin, J.; Goepfert, H. The development and validation of a dyspha-gia-specific quality-of-life questionnaire for patients with head and neck cancer: The M. D. Anderson dysphagia inventory. *Arch. Otolaryngol. Head Neck Surg.* **2001**, *127*, 870–876.
26. Cabanillas, R.; Rodrigo, J.P.; Llorente, J.L.; Suárez, V.; Ortega, P.; Suárez, C. Functional outcomes of transoral laser surgery of supraglottic carcinoma compared with a transcervical approach. *Head Neck* **2004**, *26*, 653–659. [CrossRef]

Article

Association between Temporomandibular Joint Disorder and Weight Changes: A Longitudinal Follow-Up Study Using a National Health Screening Cohort

So Young Kim [1,†], Dae Myoung Yoo [2,†], Soo-Hwan Byun [3], Chanyang Min [2,4], Ji Hee Kim [5], Mi Jung Kwon [6], Joo-Hee Kim [7] and Hyo Geun Choi [2,8,*]

1. Department of Otorhinolaryngology-Head & Neck Surgery, CHA Bundang Medical Center, CHA University, Seongnam 13496, Korea; sossi81@hanmail.net
2. Hallym Data Science Laboratory, Hallym University College of Medicine, Anyang 14068, Korea; ydm1285@naver.com (D.M.Y.); joicemin@naver.com (C.M.)
3. Department of Oral & Maxillofacial Surgery, Dentistry, Hallym University College of Medicine, Anyang 14068, Korea; purheit@daum.net
4. Graduate School of Public Health, Seoul National University, Seoul 08826, Korea
5. Department of Neurosurgery, Hallym University College of Medicine, Anyang 14068, Korea; kimjihee.ns@gmail.com
6. Department of Pathology, Hallym University College of Medicine, Anyang 14068, Korea; mulank@hanmail.net
7. Division of Pulmonary, Allergy, and Critical Care Medicine, Department of Medicine, Hallym University College of Medicine, Anyang 14068, Korea; luxjhee@gmail.com
8. Department of Otorhinolaryngology-Head & Neck Surgery, Hallym University College of Medicine, Anyang 14068, Korea
* Correspondence: pupen@naver.com
† These two authors are equally contributed to this work.

Abstract: This study aimed to investigate BMI changes following a temporomandibular joint disorder (TMJD) diagnosis. The Korean National Health Insurance Service-Health Screening Cohort from 2002 to 2015 was used. In Study I, 1808 patients with TMJD (TMJD I) were matched with 7232 participants in comparison group I. The change in BMI was compared between the TMJD I and comparison I groups for 1 year. In study II, 1621 patients with TMJD (TMJD II) were matched with 6484 participants in comparison group II participants. The change in BMI was compared between the TMJD II and comparison II groups for 2 years. In Study I, the BMI change was not associated with TMJD. In Study II, the BMI change was associated with TMJD in the interaction of the linear mixed model ($p = 0.003$). The estimated value (EV) of the linear mixed model was -0.082. The interaction was significant in women < 60 years old, women ≥ 60 years old, and the obese I category. TMJD was not associated with BMI changes after 1–2 years in the overall population. In women and obese patients, TMJD was associated with a decrease in BMI after 2 years.

Keywords: temporomandibular joint disorder; obesity; risk factors; cohort studies

1. Introduction

Temporomandibular disorder (TMD) is a group of disorders that includes temporomandibular joint (TMJ) pain and dysfunction. It might originate from changes in the structure and function of the TMJ, masticator muscle, and osseous structure [1]. It is the most common orofacial pain, and its prevalence is ~20% of the general population [2]. The peak onset age of TMD was reported to be between 20 and 40 years old and to mainly present in women [3]. In Korea, 11.8% of the general population experiences TMD [4]. The risk factors for TMD have been reported to be obesity, occlusion abnormalities, bruxism, trauma, osteoporosis, stress, anxiety, and depression [5,6]. Temporomandibular joint disorder (TMJD) is one of the common etiologies of TMD, and is prevalent in older population without gender preference [7].

The common symptoms of TMD are pain and difficulty during mastication [1]. It results in problems in the oral preparatory phase with solid (33%) and liquid (28%) swallowing [8]. TMD can cause headaches, neck pain, body pain, and dietary problems [9,10]. It has also been reported that TMD can cause weight loss (26%) [8]. However, this last study was not compared with an appropriate comparison group and studied in a limited population (n = 178) using only a self-report survey [8].

We hypothesized that TMJD might be associated with weight loss, as it is closely associated to mastication function. However, this relationship had not previously been evaluated using rigorous methods. We evaluated this association using health check-up data that were objectively measured and compared the data with the matched comparison participants using a large population-based cohort.

2. Materials and Methods

2.1. Study Population

This study was approved by the Ethics Committee of Hallym University (2019-10-023). The Institutional Review Board waived the requirement of written informed consent. This study used the Korean National Health Insurance Service–Health Screening Cohort data [11].

2.2. Definition of Temporomandibular Joint Disorder (Independent Variable)

The participants had been diagnosed under the diagnostic code for TMJD (ICD-10: K07.6 (temporomandibular joint disorders)). Participants who had histories of two or more clinical visits presenting with TMJD were included [9,12].

2.3. Definition of Weight Change (Dependent Variable)

In study I, BMI change safter one year from the TMJD diagnosis were followed up. In study II, BMI changes after two years from the diagnosis of TMJD were followed up (Study II).

2.4. Participant Selection

From total cohort data from 2002–2015 with 514,866 participants, 4627 TMJD participants were enrolled. TMJD participants who did not provide follow-up data (n = 1480) were excluded. From the identical total cohort data, comparison participants who had no history of TMJD were selected (n = 510,239). Comparison participants who had a history of TMJD were excluded (n = 6659). The comparison participants were randomly selected to prevent selection bias. The 1917 comparison participants provided 1-year follow-up data. The 1722 comparison participants provided 2-year follow-up data. A total of 492 comparison participants provided both one-year and two-year follow-up data.

In Study I, 99 TMJD participants were excluded due to a diagnosed history of TMJD before 2002 (washout periods). TMJD participants who did not have BMI records were excluded (n = 7). TMJD participants were 1:4 matched with comparison participants for age, sex, income, region of residence, and obesity. The index date of each TMJD participant was defined as the time of diagnosis of TMJD. The index date of the comparison participants was matched with their matched TMJD participants. Three TMJD participants and 496,348 comparison participants were excluded due to unmatched data. Finally, 1808 participants in the TMJD I group and 7232 participants in the comparison I group were selected (Figure 1).

In Study II, TMJD participants who had been followed up for 2 or more years were selected. The TMD participants and their matched comparison II participants were enrolled with identical inclusion and exclusion criteria. There were 64 patients who were diagnosed with TMJD before 2002 and 36 patients who did not have BMI records. These TMJD patients were excluded from the TMJD II group. Finally, 1621 TMJD II participants and 6484 comparison II participants were enrolled (Figure 1).

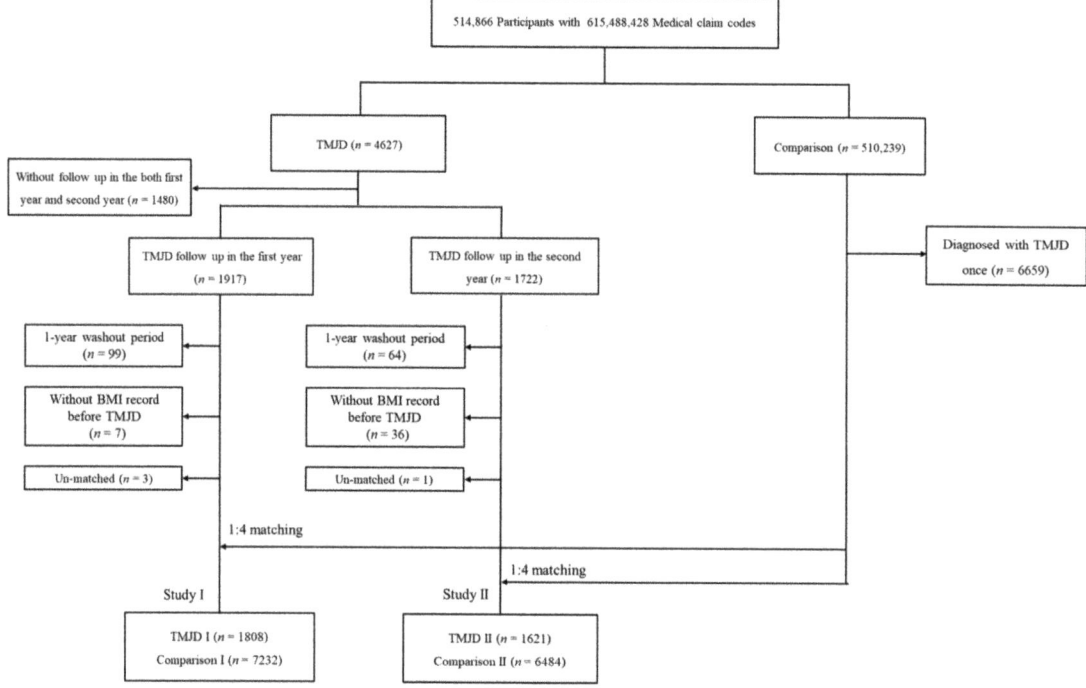

Figure 1. A schematic illustration of the participant selection process that was used in the present study. Of a total of 514,866 participants, 4627 TMJD participants were selected. Among them, we excluded participants without histories of first- or second-year follow-up records (n = 1480). Then, participants were categorized as TMJD I with a first year of follow-up (n = 1917) and TMJD II with a second year of follow-up (1722). A total of 492 TMJD participants were included in both groups. After the exclusion of 1 year of wash out, participants without BMI records, and unmatched participants, TMJD participants were 1:4 matched with comparison participants.

2.5. Covariates

The 40 years and older study population was divided into 10 age groups with 5-year intervals. Level of income was divided into 5 classes [13]. Regions of residence was divided into urban and rural areas [11]. Participants' histories of tobacco smoking and alcohol consumption were surveyed. Participants' systolic blood pressure, diastolic blood pressure, fasting blood glucose, and total cholesterol levels were measured [11]. The Charlson Comorbidity Index (CCI) was calculated as a continuous variable (between 0 (no comorbidities) and 29 (multiple comorbidities)). BMI (kg/m^2) was classified as underweight (<18.5), normal ($\geq$18.5 to <23), overweight ($\geq$23 to <25), obese I ($\geq$25 to <30), or obese II ($\geq$30) [14].

2.6. Statistical Analyses

The chi-square test was used to calculate the differences in the rates of general characteristics.

Paired t-tests were used to analyze the differences in weight pre- and post-TMJD diagnosis. A linear mixed model was used to analyze the interaction and estimated value (EV). The independent variables of age, sex, income, region of residence, TMJD, and time of measurement were used as the fixed effects. BMI, systolic blood pressure, diastolic blood pressure, fasting blood glucose, total cholesterol level, smoking status, alcohol consumption, and CCI scores were used as random effects. A first-order autoregressive model was selected as the repeated covariance type, which considered the correlation of each participant's iteration. The statistical analysis model of the linear mixed model is as follows.

$$Y_i = X_{i1}\beta_1 + \ldots + X_{ip}\beta_p + Z_{i1}u_i + \ldots + Z_{iq}u_q + e_i, \text{ for all } i = 1,\ldots,n$$

where $Y = (Y_1,\ldots, Y_n)'$, X is the $n \times p$ matrix of covariates with fixed effects $\beta = (\beta_1,\ldots, \beta_p)'$, Z is the $n \times q$ matrix of covariates with random effects, $u = (u_1,\ldots, u_q)' \sim N(0, \tau I_q)$, and the residual error vector $e = (e_1,\ldots, e_n)' \sim N(0, \tau I_n)$.

Subgroup analyses were conducted according to age and sex (<60 years and ≥60 years; men and women) and by obesity status (underweight, normal, overweight, obese I, obese II).

Two-tailed analyses were conducted. Statistical significance was defined as $p < 0.05/2$ to avoid type I error caused by the comparison of two studies. SAS version 9.4 (SAS Institute Inc., Cary, NC, USA) was used.

3. Results

The general characteristics of age, sex, income, and region of residence were exactly the same between the TMJD and comparison groups in both Study I and Study II due to matching (Table 1).

Table 1. General characteristics of participants.

Characteristics	Study I					Study II			
	Total (n)	TMJD I (n, %)	Total (n)	Comparison I (n, %)	p-Value	Total (n)	TMJD II (n, %)	Total (n)	Comparison II (n, %)	p-Value
Age (years)					1.000					1.000
40–44	1808	66 (3.7)	7232	264 (3.7)		1621	64 (4.0)	6484	256 (4.0)	
45–49	1808	239 (13.2)	7232	956 (13.2)		1621	199 (12.3)	6484	796 (12.3)	
50–54	1808	326 (18.0)	7232	1304 (18.0)		1621	358 (22.1)	6484	1432 (22.1)	
55–59	1808	359 (19.9)	7232	1436 (19.9)		1621	265 (16.4)	6484	1060 (16.4)	
60–64	1808	228 (12.6)	7232	912 (12.6)		1621	192 (11.8)	6484	768 (11.8)	
65–69	1808	247 (13.7)	7232	988 (13.7)		1621	209 (12.9)	6484	836 (12.9)	
70–74	1808	188 (10.4)	7232	752 (10.4)		1621	221 (13.6)	6484	884 (13.6)	
75–79	1808	131 (7.3)	7232	524 (7.3)		1621	80 (4.9)	6484	320 (4.9)	
80–84	1808	21 (1.2)	7232	84 (1.2)		1621	30 (1.9)	6484	120 (1.9)	
85+	1808	3 (0.2)	7232	12 (0.2)		1621	3 (0.2)	6484	12 (0.2)	
Sex					1.000					1.000
Male	1808	849 (47.0)	7232	3396 (47.0)		1621	737 (45.5)	6484	2948 (45.5)	
Female	1808	959 (53.0)	7232	3836 (53.0)		1621	884 (54.5)	6484	3536 (54.5)	
Income					1.000					1.000
1 (lowest)	1808	283 (15.7)	7232	1132 (15.7)		1621	244 (15.1)	6484	976 (15.1)	
2	1808	252 (13.9)	7232	1008 (13.9)		1621	231 (14.3)	6484	924 (14.3)	
3	1808	281 (15.5)	7232	1124 (15.5)		1621	277 (17.1)	6484	1108 (17.1)	
4	1808	375 (20.7)	7232	1500 (20.7)		1621	340 (21.0)	6484	1360 (21.0)	
5 (highest)	1808	617 (34.1)	7232	2468 (34.1)		1621	529 (32.6)	6484	2116 (32.6)	
Region of residence					1.000					1.000
Urban	1808	740 (40.9)	7232	2960 (40.9)		1621	675 (41.6)	6484	2700 (41.6)	
Rural	1808	1068 (59.1)	7232	4272 (59.1)		1621	946 (58.4)	6484	3784 (58.4)	
Obesity †					1.000					1.000
Underweight	1808	43 (2.4)	7232	172 (2.4)		1621	38 (2.3)	6484	152 (2.3)	
Normal	1808	725 (40.1)	7232	2900 (40.1)		1621	637 (39.3)	6484	2548 (39.3)	
Overweight	1808	529 (29.3)	7232	2116 (29.3)		1621	472 (29.1)	6484	1888 (29.1)	
Obese I	1808	474 (26.2)	7232	1896 (26.2)		1621	445 (27.5)	6484	1780 (27.5)	
Obese II	1808	37 (2.1)	7232	148 (2.1)		1621	29 (1.8)	6484	116 (1.8)	
Smoking status					0.036 *					0.002 *
Nonsmoker	1808	1346 (74.5)	7232	5357 (74.1)		1621	1250 (77.1)	6484	4820 (74.3)	
Past smoker	1808	228 (12.6)	7232	801 (11.1)		1621	178 (11.0)	6484	671 (10.4)	
Current smoker	1808	234 (12.9)	7232	1074 (14.9)		1621	193 (11.9)	6484	993 (15.3)	
Alcohol consumption					0.572					0.879
<1 time a week	1808	1319 (73.0)	7232	5228 (72.3)		1621	1197 (73.8)	6484	4800 (74.0)	
≥1 time a week	1808	489 (27.1)	7232	2004 (27.7)		1621	424 (26.2)	6484	1684 (26.0)	

Table 1. Cont.

Characteristics	Total (n)	Study I TMJD I (n, %)	Total (n)	Comparison I (n, %)	p-Value	Total (n)	Study II TMJD II (n, %)	Total (n)	Comparison II (n, %)	p-Value
Systolic blood pressure					0.002 *					0.007 *
<120 mmHg	1808	629 (34.8)	7232	2338 (32.3)		1621	561 (34.6)	6484	2078 (32.1)	
120–139 mmHg	1808	900 (49.8)	7232	3531 (48.8)		1621	787 (48.6)	6484	3100 (47.8)	
≥140 mmHg	1808	279 (15.4)	7232	1363 (18.9)		1621	273 (16.8)	6484	1306 (20.1)	
Diastolic blood pressure					0.002 *					0.005 *
<80 mmHg	1808	930 (51.4)	7232	3524 (48.7)		1621	839 (51.8)	6484	3079 (47.5)	
80–89 mmHg	1808	647 (35.8)	7232	2545 (35.2)		1621	550 (33.9)	6484	2331 (36.0)	
≥90 mmHg	1808	231 (12.8)	7232	1163 (16.1)		1621	232 (14.3)	6484	1074 (16.6)	
Fasting blood glucose					0.188					0.381
<100 mg/dL	1808	1201 (66.4)	7232	4746 (65.6)		1621	1104 (68.1)	6484	4359 (67.2)	
100–125 mg/dL	1808	497 (27.5)	7232	1957 (27.1)		1621	411 (25.4)	6484	1636 (25.2)	
≥126 mg/dL	1808	110 (6.1)	7232	529 (7.3)		1621	106 (6.5)	6484	489 (7.5)	
Total cholesterol					0.016 *					0.510
<200 mg/dL	1808	999 (55.3)	7232	3788 (52.4)		1621	870 (53.7)	6484	3377 (52.1)	
200–239 mg/dL	1808	607 (33.6)	7232	2470 (34.2)		1621	544 (33.6)	6484	2261 (34.9)	
≥240 mg/dL	1808	202 (11.2)	7232	974 (13.5)		1621	207 (12.8)	6484	846 (13.1)	
CCI score					0.562					0.297
0	1808	1286 (71.1)	7232	5221 (72.2)		1621	1162 (71.7)	6484	4737 (73.1)	
1	1808	259 (14.3)	7232	974 (13.5)		1621	225 (13.9)	6484	867 (13.4)	
2	1808	143 (7.9)	7232	526 (7.3)		1621	131 (8.1)	6484	434 (6.7)	
3	1808	52 (2.9)	7232	245 (3.4)		1621	50 (3.1)	6484	205 (3.2)	
≥4	1808	68 (3.8)	7232	266 (3.7)		1621	53 (3.3)	6484	241 (3.7)	

Abbreviations: CCI, Charlson comorbidity index; TMJD, Temporomandibular joint disorder. * Chi-square test; significance was defined as $p < 0.05$. † Obesity (BMI, body mass index, kg/m^2) was categorized as underweight (<18.5), normal (≥18.5 to <23), overweight (≥23 to <25), obese I (≥25 to <30), and obese II (≥30).

The paired t-test did not show differences between the pre- and post-TMJD 1-year records of the participants in the TMJD I and comparison I groups (Table 2). The interaction in the linear mixed model did not reach statistical significance in Study I. The decrease in BMI was significant in the TMJD I group of men aged <60 years, but this change was not significant in the interaction model.

Table 2. Differences in mean BMI between pre- and 1-year-post-study of TMJD in Study I according to age and sex.

Characteristics	TMJD I			Comparison I			Interaction ‡	Linear Mixed Model ¶	
	Previous (Mean, SD)	Post 1yr (Mean, SD)	p-Value	Previous (Mean, SD)	Post 1yr (Mean, SD)	p-Value	p-Value	EV §	p-Value
Total participants (n = 9040)	23.58 ± 2.83	23.58 ± 2.83	0.957	23.62 ± 2.84	23.62 ± 2.89	0.979	0.769	−0.014	0.850
Age 40–60 years old, men (n = 2365)	23.92 ± 2.54	24.04 ± 2.54	0.010 *	23.98 ± 2.66	24.02 ± 2.67	0.154	0.146	0.044	0.736
Age 40–60 years old, women (n = 2585)	23.45 ± 3.09	23.49 ± 3.09	0.374	23.44 ± 2.92	23.47 ± 2.95	0.394	0.799	0.055	0.698
Age ≥60 years old, men (n = 1880)	23.23 ± 2.76	23.06 ± 2.62	0.032	23.28 ± 2.78	23.22 ± 2.83	0.092	0.208	−0.135	0.389
Age ≥60 years old, women (n = 2210)	23.67 ± 2.84	23.61 ± 2.91	0.397	23.73 ± 2.94	23.72 ± 3.02	0.668	0.468	−0.069	0.656

Abbreviations: CCI, Charlson Comorbidity Index; EV, estimated value; TMJD, temporomandibular joint disorders. * Paired t-test; significance was defined as $p < 0.05/2$. ‡ Interaction effects between time and group. § Estimated value of the linear mixed model for TMJD I group based on the comparison I group. ¶ Fixed effects were age, sex, income, region of residence, TMJD, and time of measurement. Random effects were systolic blood pressure, diastolic blood pressure, fasting blood glucose, total cholesterol, smoking, alcohol consumption, and CCI score.

In the subgroup analyses according to obesity status, the change in weight was significant in both the TMJD I and comparison I groups, except for the overweight group (Table 3). In the underweight/normal weight category, the BMIs of the participants in both the TMJD I and comparison I groups increased. In the obese I category, the BMIs of the participants in the TMJD I group decreased and those in participants in comparison I group increased. In the obese II category, the BMIs of the participants in both the TMJD I and comparison I groups decreased. However, none of these changes were statistically significant in the interaction model.

Table 3. Differences in mean BMI between pre- and 1-year-post-study of TMJD in TMJD I and the comparison I group according to obesity.

Characteristics	TMJD I			Comparison I			Interaction ‡	Linear Mixed Model ¶	
	Previous (Mean, SD)	Post 1 Year (Mean, SD)	p-Value	Previous (Mean, SD)	Post 1 Year (Mean, SD)	p-Value	p-Value	EV §	p-Value
Underweight (n = 215)	17.55 ± 0.80	17.99 ± 1.09	0.008 *	17.57 ± 0.79	18.05 ± 1.46	<0.001 *	0.810	−0.046	0.807
Normal (n = 3625)	21.26 ± 1.16	21.49 ± 1.55	<0.001 *	21.26 ± 1.17	21.46 ± 1.63	<0.001 *	0.649	0.042	0.465
Overweight (n = 2645)	23.96 ± 0.56	23.91 ± 1.19	0.254	24.01 ± 0.57	23.98 ± 1.29	0.334	0.584	−0.068	0.154
Obese I (n = 2370)	26.58 ± 1.19	26.34 ± 1.82	<0.001 *	26.73 ± 1.26	26.47 ± 1.74	<0.001 *	0.785	−0.108	0.165
Obese II (n = 185)	31.99 ± 2.45	30.72 ± 3.04	0.007 *	31.52 ± 1.54	30.75 ± 2.34	<0.001 *	0.165	−0.087	0.821

Abbreviations: CCI, Charlson Comorbidity Index; EV, estimated value; TMJD, temporomandibular joint disorders. * Paired t-test; significance was defined as $p < 0.05/2$. ‡ Interaction effects between time and group. § Estimated value of the linear mixed model for the TMJD I group based on the comparison I group. ¶ Fixed effects were age, sex, income, region of residence, TMJD, and time of measurement. Random effects were systolic blood pressure, diastolic blood pressure, fasting blood glucose, total cholesterol, smoking, alcohol consumption, and CCI score.

The paired t-test did not show differences in the pre- and post-TMJD 2-year records among all participants in the TMJD II and comparison II groups (Table 4). On the other hand, the interaction in the linear mixed model reached statistical significance ($p = 0.003$), and the EV of the linear mixed model was −0.082. A decrease in BMI was found in the TMJD II group in women ≥ 60 years old, while an increase in BMI was observed in the comparison II group in men < 60 years old and women < 60 years old. The interaction was significant in women < 60 years old and women ≥ 60 years old. The EV was −0.109 for women < 60 years old and −0.272 in women ≥ 60 years old.

Table 4. Differences in mean BMI between pre- and 2-year-post-study of TMJD in Study II according to age and sex.

Characteristics	TMJD II			Comparison II			Interaction ‡	Linear Mixed Model ¶	
	Previous (Mean, SD)	Post 2 Years (Mean, SD)	p-Value	Previous (Mean, SD)	Post 2 Years (Mean, SD)	p-Value	p-Value	EV §	p-Value
Total participants (n = 8105)	23.70 ± 2.96	23.62 ± 2.84	0.064	23.69 ± 2.82	23.72 ± 2.90	0.148	0.003 †	−0.082	0.294
Age 40–60 years, men (n = 2090)	24.13 ± 2.68	24.21 ± 2.55	0.156	24.07 ± 2.65	24.14 ± 2.70	0.023 *	0.879	0.047	0.740
Age 40–60 years, women (n = 2340)	23.38 ± 3.41	23.28 ± 2.98	0.343	23.28 ± 2.84	23.42 ± 2.87	<0.001 *	0.003 †	−0.109	0.458
Age ≥60 years, men (n = 1595)	23.36 ± 2.58	23.33 ± 2.83	0.763	23.39 ± 2.62	23.33 ± 2.77	0.110	0.963	0.023	0.888
Age ≥60 years, women (n = 2080)	23.90 ± 2.87	23.64 ± 2.88	0.001 *	24.00 ± 3.02	23.93 ± 3.14	0.109	0.023†	−0.272	0.098

Abbreviations: CCI, Charlson Comorbidity Index; EV, estimated value; TMJD, temporomandibular joint disorders. * Paired t-test; significance was defined as $p < 0.05/2$. † Linear mixed model; significance was defined as $p < 0.05/2$. ‡ Interaction effects between time and group. § Estimated value of the linear mixed model for the TMJD II group based on the comparison II group. ¶ Fixed effects were age, sex, income, region of residence, TMJD, and time of measurement. Random effects were systolic blood pressure, diastolic blood pressure, fasting blood glucose, total cholesterol, smoking, alcohol consumption, and CCI score.

In the subgroup analyses according to obesity status, an increase in BMI was observed in underweight/normal weight individuals in the TMJD II and comparison II groups (Table 5). A decrease in BMI was found in obese individuals in the TMJD II and comparison II groups. The interaction model was significant in the obese I category, and its EV was −0.200.

Table 5. Differences in mean BMI between pre- and 2-year-post-study of TMJD in TMJD II and comparison II group according to obesity.

Characteristics	TMJD II			Comparison II			Interaction ‡	Linear Mixed Model ¶	
	Previous (Mean, SD)	Post 1 Year (Mean, SD)	p-Value	Previous (Mean, SD)	Post 1 Year (Mean, SD)	p-Value	p-Value	EV §	p-Value
Underweight ($n = 190$)	17.52 ± 0.88	18.58 ± 1.86	0.003 *	17.50 ± 0.91	18.13 ± 1.72	<0.001 *	0.202	0.467	0.061
Normal ($n = 3185$)	21.39 ± 1.14	21.56 ± 1.51	<0.001 *	21.38 ± 1.14	21.63 ± 1.68	<0.001 *	0.151	−0.071	0.248
Overweight ($n = 2360$)	23.96 ± 0.57	23.90 ± 1.59	0.355	23.98 ± 0.57	23.94 ± 1.40	0.292	0.574	−0.039	0.488
Obese I ($n = 2225$)	26.66 ± 1.25	26.24 ± 1.87	<0.001 *	26.69 ± 1.25	26.45 ± 1.88	<0.001 *	0.010 †	−0.200	0.017 †
Obese II ($n = 145$)	33.08 ± 6.27	30.84 ± 4.10	0.139	31.96 ± 3.26	31.33 ± 2.83	0.057	0.095	−0.541	0.460

Abbreviations: CCI, Charlson Comorbidity Index; EV, estimated value; TMJD, temporomandibular joint disorders. * Paired t-test; significance was defined as $p < 0.05/2$. † Linear mixed model; significance was defined as $p < 0.05/2$. ‡ Interaction effects between time and group. § Estimated value of the linear mixed model for the TMJD II group based on the comparison II group. ¶ Fixed effects were age, sex, income, region of residence, TMJD, and time of measurement. Random effects were systolic blood pressure, diastolic blood pressure, fasting blood glucose, total cholesterol, smoking, alcohol consumption, and CCI score.

4. Discussion

It was found that the change in BMI was significant only in Study II, which measured the 2-year change in patients with TMJD in the present study. A decrease in BMI was observed in the TMJD II group compared with the comparison II group only in women and the obese I category. This association was not found in any of the subgroups of Study I, which had a 1-year follow-up. This is the first study that reports the change in BMI in TMJD participants compared to matched comparison participants.

We believe this change in BMI is clinically meaningful, even though statistical significance was observed only in the women and obese I subgroups with the 2-year follow-up. The BMI change over 1 or 2 years was not significant in most of the subgroups, and the change in BMI was very small. As this study enrolled a large number of participants, statistical significance was detected with these minimal changes in BMI. In this study, among the statistically significant values, the largest EV was −0.272. This means that the BMIs of the participants in the TMJD group decreased by −0.272 compared to those of participants in of the comparison group. If the height of a participant were 170 cm, their BMI would change by −0.78 kg in 2 years.

The association of TMD with BMI has been suggested in several prior studies with differing results [5,15–18]. In a cross-sectional study, TMD was associated with low BMI in women (adjusted odds ratio (aOR) = 1.44, 95% confidence interval (95% CI) = 1.09–1.93, $p = 0.037$) [5]. However, other cross-sectional studies demonstrated no association between BMI and TMD in adolescents [15] or the general population [16]. On the other hand, overweight (BMI ≥ 25) was associated with frequent pain-associated TMD symptoms among Finnish conscripts (aOR = 1.23, 95% CI = 1.01–1.49) [18]. Another cross-sectional study in an adult population suggested an association of TMD with obesity in a univariate analysis. These differing observed associations between TMD and weight loss may originate from the limited numbers of participants in the above studies. Previously, few studies reported such an association compared with comparison groups. In addition, the potential effects of the aging process on weight loss could not be excluded in previous studies, because they did not have comparison participants who matched for age and BMI. As follow-up durations were not defined in most prior studies, the temporal association between TMD and weight loss could not be estimated.

TMJD could be associated with decreased BMI due to changes in eating behaviors and stress factors associated with TMJD. Patients with TMD may have weakened biting force, which impairs masticatory movement [19]. The pain of TMJ was reported to affect dietary intake, which leads to the avoidance of specific foods, such as meat and apples [20]. In addition, patients with TMD showed a higher rate of mental stress [5]. Mental stress was reported to delay the gastrointestinal transit time and peak glucose response, which decreased the appetite and dietary intake [21]. Mastication difficulties, pain, and psychological stress could decrease a person's dietary intake, which may result in a decreased BMI in patients with TMD. Because obesity was suggested to be one of the factors associated with TMD, the present study analyzed the impact of TMD on BMI changes according to different BMI groups. As a result, the obese I population showed an association of TMD with decreased BMI. Compared with male subgroups, female subgroups demonstrated decreased BMI associated with TMJD in this study. Similar to the present result, a previous study also reported a sex-specific association of TMD with decreased BMI [5]. They supposed that a higher susceptibility to psychological stress and anxiety associated with TMD in women may be linked with a decreased BMI [5].

In the overall population and other subgroups, TMJD was not associated with BMI changes in the present study. Several explanations could support the present results. First, the decreased dietary intake could be compensated by the substitution of foods by patients with TMJD. A survey described the modifications of diet in patients with TMD [22]. Approximately 77.6% (66/85) of TMD patients modified their diet, including by cutting food into smaller pieces (71.8% [61/85]), softening (42.4% [36/85]), and mashing (40% [34/85]) their food [22]. By these efforts, the potential risk of nutritional deficits could be prevented in patients with TMJD. Second, a decrease in BMI could relieve the pain and other symptoms of TMJD, which alleviates dietary disturbances in TMJD patients. Third, the contribution of TMJD to BMI changes was not considerable, and many other factors could mediate the link between TMJD and BMI changes. For instance, a previous study reported that the association of TMD with obesity was not evident after adjusting for sex and other comorbidities, such as headaches and obstructive sleep apnea [17]. As the present study comprehensively adjusted for potential confounders, that could explain why the association of TMJD with BMI changes was not statistically significant.

The present study used a large nationwide cohort population. Many comparison participants were matched for age, sex, income, region of residence, and obesity status, and were randomly selected. The variables were reliable and were collected from national health insurance and health check-up data. Participants' past medical histories were based on diagnostic codes, and laboratory measures were used for the levels of blood pressure, blood glucose, and total cholesterol. The accuracy of BMI data could be guaranteed by objective measures during health check-ups. In addition, the duration of follow-up was classified into 1 year and 2 years, so that we could assess the sensitivity of the association of TMJD with weight loss. To minimize the bias due to multiple comparisons, the Bonferroni correction was conducted. However, the long-term effects of TMJD on weight loss could not be evaluated in the present cohort data. To compensate for the short follow-up duration of this study, two independent studies were conducted with 1-year and 2-year follow-up durations. This study was based on health check-up data, thus selection bias cannot be excluded. Some information about our cohort was not accessible, which could induce information bias. The severity of TMJD was heterogeneous, and the treatment histories of patients with TMJD were not available in this study. Because this study was based on diagnostic code ICD10, the etiology of TMJD could not be isolated. TMJD could be mixed with TMD. However, TMD is more common in children and adolescents [23]. On the other hand, TMJD was more common in the elderly population in our study and was associated with TMJ degeneration [7]. Although many comorbidities, anthropometric data, and lifestyle factors were adjusted, confounders, such as nutritional factors, may have remained. Last, a detailed etiology for weight loss could not be isolated in the present data.

5. Conclusions

Patients with TMJD did not show more changes in BMI than comparison participants in the overall population. A decrease in BMI associated with TMJD was observed in a subpopulation of women and obese patients with a 2-year follow-up duration.

Author Contributions: H.G.C. designed the study; D.M.Y., C.M., S.-H.B. and H.G.C. analyzed the data; S.Y.K., J.H.K., M.J.K., J.-H.K. and H.G.C. drafted and revised the paper; and H.G.C. drew the figures. All authors have read and agreed to the published version of the manuscript.

Funding: This work was supported in part by research grants (NRF-2018-R1D1A1A02085328 and 2021-R1C1C100498611) from the National Research Foundation (NRF) of Korea and Hallym University Research Fund (HURF). The APC was funded by NRF-2021-R1C1C100498611.

Institutional Review Board Statement: The Ethics Committee of Hallym University (2014-I148) approved the use of the data. The need for written informed consent was waived by the Institutional Review Board.

Informed Consent Statement: Written informed consent was waived by the Institutional Review Board.

Data Availability Statement: Releasing of the data by the researcher is not legally permitted. All data are available from the database of the Korea Center for Disease Control and Prevention. The Korea Center for Disease Control and Prevention allows data access, at a certain cost, for any researcher who promises to follow the stipulated code of research ethics. The data of this article can be downloaded from the website after agreeing to follow the code.

Conflicts of Interest: The authors declare no conflict of interest.

References

1. Gilheaney, Ó.; Stassen, L.F.; Walshe, M. The epidemiology, nature, and impact of eating and swallowing problems in adults presenting with temporomandibular disorders. *Cranio* **2020**, *2020*, 1–9. [CrossRef] [PubMed]
2. Dworkin, S.F.; Huggins, K.H.; LeResche, L.; Von Korff, M.; Howard, J.; Truelove, E.; Sommers, E. Epidemiology of Signs and Symptoms in Temporomandibular Disorders: Clinical Signs in Cases and Controls. *J. Am. Dent. Assoc.* **1990**, *120*, 273–281. [CrossRef]
3. Liu, F.; Steinkeler, A. Epidemiology, Diagnosis, and Treatment of Temporomandibular Disorders. *Dent. Clin. N. Am.* **2013**, *57*, 465–479. [CrossRef] [PubMed]
4. Song, H.-S.; Shin, J.-S.; Lee, J.; Lee, Y.J.; Kim, M.-R.; Cho, J.-H.; Kim, K.-W.; Park, Y.; Park, S.-Y.; Kim, S.; et al. Association between temporomandibular disorders, chronic diseases, and ophthalmologic and otolaryngologic disorders in Korean adults: A cross-sectional study. *PLoS ONE* **2018**, *13*, e0191336. [CrossRef] [PubMed]
5. Rhim, E.; Han, K.; Yun, K.-I. Association between temporomandibular disorders and obesity. *J. Cranio-Maxillofac. Surg.* **2016**, *44*, 1003–1007. [CrossRef]
6. Chisnoiu, A.M.; Picos, A.M.; Popa, S.; Chisnoiu, P.D.; Lascu, L.; Picos, A.; Chisnoiu, R. Factors involved in the etiology of temporomandibular disorders—A literature review. *Med. Pharm. Rep.* **2015**, *88*, 473–478. [CrossRef]
7. Yadav, S.; Yang, Y.; Dutra, E.H.; Robinson, J.L.; Wadhwa, S. Temporomandibular Joint Disorders in Older Adults. *J. Am. Geriatr. Soc.* **2018**, *66*, 1213–1217. [CrossRef]
8. Gilheaney, Ó.; Stassen, L.F.; Walshe, M. Prevalence, Nature, and Management of Oral Stage Dysphagia in Adults With Temporomandibular Joint Disorders: Findings From an Irish Cohort. *J. Oral Maxillofac. Surg.* **2018**, *76*, 1665–1676. [CrossRef]
9. Byun, S.-H.; Min, C.; Yoo, D.-M.; Yang, B.-E.; Choi, H.-G. Increased Risk of Migraine in Patients with Temporomandibular Disorder: A Longitudinal Follow-Up Study Using a National Health Screening Cohort. *Diagnostics* **2020**, *10*, 724. [CrossRef]
10. Ohrbach, R.; Fillingim, R.B.; Mulkey, F.; Gonzalez, Y.; Gordon, S.; Gremillion, H.; Lim, P.-F.; Ribeiro-Dasilva, M.; Greenspan, J.D.; Knott, C.; et al. Clinical findings and pain symptoms as potential risk factors for chronic TMD: Descriptive data and empirically identified domains from the OPPERA case-control study. *J. Pain* **2011**, *12*, T27–T45. [CrossRef]
11. Kim, S.Y.; Min, C.; Oh, D.J.; Choi, H.G. Tobacco Smoking and Alcohol Consumption Are Related to Benign Parotid Tumor: A Nested Case-Control Study Using a National Health Screening Cohort. *Clin. Exp. Otorhinolaryngol.* **2019**, *12*, 412–419. [CrossRef]
12. Byun, S.-H.; Min, C.; Choi, H.-G.; Hong, S.J. Increased Risk of Temporomandibular Joint Disorder in Patients with Rheumatoid Arthritis: A Longitudinal Follow-Up Study. *J. Clin. Med.* **2020**, *9*, 3005. [CrossRef]
13. Kim, S.Y.; Min, C.; Yoo, D.M.; Chang, J.; Lee, H.-J.; Park, B.; Choi, H.G. Hearing Impairment Increases Economic Inequality. *Clin. Exp. Otorhinolaryngol.* **2021**, *14*, 278–286. [CrossRef]
14. WHO, I. IOTF. The Asia-Pacific Perspective. Redefining Obesity and Its Treatment. In *Obesity: Preventing and Managing the Global Epidemic*; WHO: Geneva, Switzerland, 2000.
15. Jordani, P.C.; Campi, L.B.; Braido, G.V.V.; Fernandes, G.; Visscher, C.M.; Gonçalves, D. Obesity, sedentarism and TMD-pain in adolescents. *J. Oral Rehabil.* **2019**, *46*, 460–467. [CrossRef]
16. Ahlberg, J.P.; Kovero, O.A.; Hurmerinta, K.A.; Zepa, I.; Nissinen, M.J.; Könönen, M.H. Maximal bite force and its association with signs and symptoms of TMD, occlusion, and body mass index in a cohort of young adults. *Cranio* **2003**, *21*, 248–252. [CrossRef]
17. Jordani, P.C.; Campi, L.; Circeli, G.Z.; Visscher, C.M.; Bigal, M.E.; Gonçalves, D. Obesity as a risk factor for temporomandibular disorders. *J. Oral Rehabil.* **2016**, *44*, 1–8. [CrossRef] [PubMed]
18. Miettinen, O.; Kämppi, A.; Tanner, T.; Anttonen, V.; Patinen, P.; Päkkilä, J.; Tjäderhane, L.; Sipilä, K. Association of Temporomandibular Disorder Symptoms with Physical Fitness among Finnish Conscripts. *Int. J. Environ. Res. Public Health* **2021**, *18*, 3032. [CrossRef]

19. Pereira, L.J.; Gavião, M.B.D.; Bonjardim, L.R.; Castelo, P.M.; Van Der Bilt, A. Muscle thickness, bite force, and craniofacial dimensions in adolescents with signs and symptoms of temporomandibular dysfunction. *Eur. J. Orthod.* **2007**, *29*, 72–78. [CrossRef] [PubMed]
20. Irving, J.; Wood, G.; Hackett, A. Does temporomandibular disorder pain dysfunction syndrome affect dietary intake? *Dent. Update* **1999**, *26*, 405–407. [CrossRef] [PubMed]
21. Wing, R.R.; Blair, E.H.; Epstein, L.H.; McDermott, M.D. Psychological stress and glucose metabolism in obese and normal-weight subjects: A possible mechanism for differences in stress-induced eating. *Health Psychol.* **1990**, *9*, 693–700. [CrossRef] [PubMed]
22. Edwards, D.C.; Bowes, C.C.; Penlington, C.; Durham, J. Temporomandibular disorders and dietary changes: A cross-sectional survey. *J. Oral Rehabil.* **2021**. [CrossRef] [PubMed]
23. Perez, C. Temporomandibular disorders in children and adolescents. *Gen. Dent.* **2018**, *66*, 51–55. [PubMed]

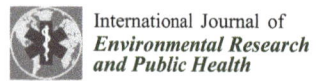

Review

Oncological Outcomes of Primary vs. Salvage OPHL Type II: A Systematic Review

Carmelo Saraniti [1], Barbara Verro [1,*], Francesco Ciodaro [2] and Francesco Galletti [2]

[1] ENT Clinic, Department of Biomedicine, Neuroscience and Advanced Diagnostic, University of Palermo, 90127 Palermo, Italy; carmelo.saraniti@unipa.it

[2] Division for Otorhinolaryngology, Department of Adult and Development Age Human Pathology "Gaetano Barresi", University of Messina, 98125 Messina, Italy; dottfciodaro@alice.it (F.C.); fgalletti@unime.it (F.G.)

* Correspondence: verrobarbara@gmail.com; Tel.: +39-327-1722-000

Abstract: *Background:* Open partial horizontal laryngectomy type II (OPHL type II) has two main aims: oncological radicality and laryngeal preservation. The aim of this review is to define and emphasize the oncological efficacy of OPHL type II, both as primary and salvage surgery, by analyzing the latest literature. *Methods:* The research was carried out on Pubmed, Scopus and Web of Science databases, by using strict keywords. Oncological outcomes were evaluated by the following parameters: overall survival, disease-specific survival, disease-free survival, local control, laryngeal preservation, local recurrence. *Results:* The review included 19 articles divided into three groups: (1) primary OPHL type II, (2) salvage OPHL type II, (3) adjuvant radiotherapy after primary OPHL type II. The articles showed excellent results as far as oncological radicality and organ preservation. *Conclusions:* This review demonstrated that OPHL type II is useful to obtain oncological radicality both as primary surgery and salvage surgery. Nevertheless, the only criterion that determined the positive outcome and efficacy of this technique is the strict selection of patient and tumor.

Keywords: otolaryngology; head and neck; laryngectomy; surgical oncology; salvage therapy

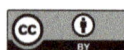

1. Introduction

Supracricoid laryngectomy, or open partial horizontal laryngectomy type II (OPHL type II), introduced in the 1950s [1] and modified by Piquet in 1974 [2], has two main aims: oncological radicality and organ preservation [3]. This surgery technique enabled researchers to limit total laryngectomy surgery and its consequences: permanent tracheostoma and loss of the natural voice [4]. In fact, in 2018, the American Society of Clinical Oncology (ASCO) recommended total laringectomy only for extensive T3 and T4a lesions to ensure better survival rate and recommended chemoradiotherapy or OPHL for locally advanced disease to ensure the greatest possible organ preservation and minimal functional impairment [5]. Particularly, T2 and selected T3 glottic and supraglottic cancers [6] are amenable with OPHL type II by removal of thyroid cartilage, true vocal folds and false vocal folds, Morgagni's sinus, pre-epiglottic space and paraglottic space. Therefore, the only preserved structures are: cricoid cartilage, one or both arytenoid cartilages, hyoid bone, and, sometimes, suprahyoid epiglottis. According to the 2014 classification by the European Laryngological Society (ELS) [7], OPHL type II can be divided into two subtypes: type IIa if suprahyoid epiglottis is preserved, so crico-hyoido-epiglottopexy (CHEP) is performed; type IIb if suprahyoid epiglottis is removed and crico-hyoidopexy (CHP) [8] is performed. The crico-arytenoid unit (CAU), composed of the crico-arytenoid joint and the underlying hemicricoid plate, guarantees the satisfactory functional outcome of this surgery; for this reason, it is fundamental to preserve at least one mobile arytenoid cartilage. Furthermore, Calearo and Bignardi, with their histological studies on the larynx and laryngeal carcinoma, have demonstrated the importance of the arytenoid for oncological radicality: in fact, thanks to the fibrous ligament on its anterior aspect, it acts as a barrier hindering the extension of the tumor to the underlying laryngeal structures [9].

Contraindications to OPHL type II are: (1) extension of the tumor to both arytenoids, to the crico-arytenoid unit or to the posterior commissure, (2) invasion of the hyoid bone, (3) extension of the tumor to the cricoid cartilage, and (4) extralaryngeal spread.

Thus, OPHL type II also serves an important role in salvage surgery after the failure of radiotherapy or TLM (transoral laser microsurgery) [10,11], reducing the use of total laryngectomy. Therefore, this partial surgery enables researchers to obtain reliable, functional and oncological results both as primary surgery and salvage surgery [12,13].

However, selection of the patients eligible for OPHL type II [10] is determined by considering localization and extension of the tumor, as well as the health and psychosocial status of the patient.

The aim of this review is to define and emphasize the oncological efficacy of OPHL type II, both as primary surgery and salvage surgery, as far as overall survival (OS), disease-specific survival (DSS), disease-free survival (DFS), local control (LC), laryngeal preservation (LP) and local recurrence (LR) are concerned, by analyzing the latest literature on this topic.

2. Materials and Methods

2.1. Search Methodology

The selection of bibliography was carried out on Pubmed, Scopus and Web of Science databases, by using the following keywords: *supracricoid laryngectomy* or *open partial laryngectomy type II* or *OPHL type II* and *oncologic outcome*. Furthermore, some articles were chosen from a bibliography of selected studies. Therefore, two independent authors (BV and CS) selected the articles: a first selection was made by reading titles and abstracts. Afterwards, the selected articles were read entirely in order to include only those that fulfilled the eligibility criteria in the study.

2.2. Eligibility Criteria

The eligibility criteria were: (1) studies that analyzed oncological outcomes exclusively of OPHL type II, (2) at least 30 patients included in the study, (3) studies that calculated at least two of the following parameters: OS, DFS, DSS, LC, LP, LR, (4) median or mean follow-up period of at least 36 months, (5) studies published from 2000 onwards.

Exclusion criteria were: (1) reviews, editorials, opinions or case reports, (2) studies that did not distinguish OS, DFS, DSS, LC, LP, LR in primary and salvage OPHL type II, (3) articles that were not written in English or Italian, (4) studies in which patients had undergone adjuvant chemotherapy.

2.3. Data Analysis

The following information was selected from chosen articles: authors, year of publication, number of included patients, follow-up duration (months), OS, DFS, DSS, LC, LP, LR. Data were collected on data spreadsheet using Microsoft Excel (version 16.47.1). OS is the time between surgery and death by any cause or last follow-up; DSS is the interval time between surgery and death from the disease; DFS is the time from surgery to tumor recurrence; LC is the length of time from surgery to relapse on the primary tumor site; LP is the interval time between OPHL to total laryngectomy; LR is the time between surgery and the first local recurrence [14,15].

3. Results

3.1. Selection and Classification of Studies

Figure 1 shows the process of selection of the studies [16]. Overall, 145 articles were selected from the systematic research. The first step included the elimination of doubles (n° 23) and, secondly, the exclusion of unrelated articles, taking into account title, abstract or language criteria (n° 90). Subsequently, 48 full studies were read independently by the two authors (BV and CS) and assessed, taking into account the eligibility criteria, including only 19 articles in the review.

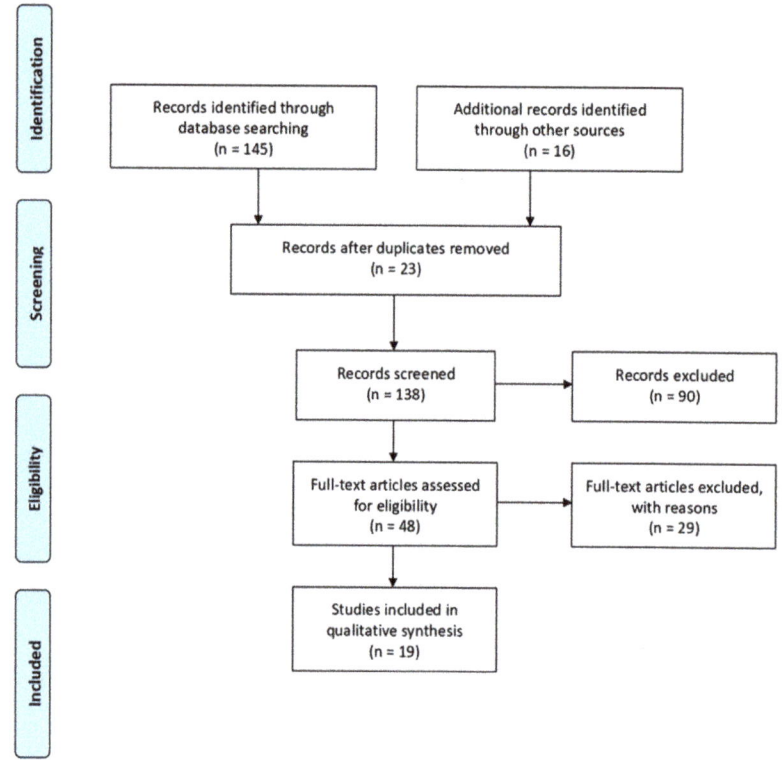

Figure 1. PRISMA 2009 Flow Diagram© of study selection process of literature (from [16]).

Afterwards, the selected articles were analyzed and grouped into three different categories: (1) primary OPHL type II, (2) salvage OPHL type II, (3) adjuvant radiotherapy after primary OPHL type II.

3.2. Primary OPHL Type II

Six primary OPHL type II [3,4,6,11,17,18] articles were selected and assessed (Table 1). Nearly all the studies included 5-year OS, corresponding to about 80% [3,4,11,17,18], except for the study by Sánchez-Cuadrado et al. [6] with a 60% 5-year OS in a sample of 41 patients. Primary OPHL type II was also efficient and resolutive considering 5-year DSS (76.7% [4] and 82.4% [18]) and LC (95.6% [3], 80% [6] and 93.94% [17]). Organ preservation, which represents the main goal of this surgery, was guaranteed by more than 85% of patients [3,6,11].

Table 1. Primary OPHL type II: characteristics of included studies.

Authors (Year of Publication)	N° Patients	pT Treated	Follow-Up	OS	DSS	DFS	LP	LC
Karasalihoglu AR et al. (2004) [3]	68	T1-T4	62 months (median)	78.6% (5 years)	93.9% (5 years)	/	89.7% (5 years)	95.6% (5 years)
Sánchez-Cuadrado I et al. (2011) [6]	41	T1-T3	43 months (median)	69% (5 years)	81% (5 years)	/	85% (5 years)	80% (5 years)
Nakayama M et al. (2013) [11]	43	T1-T4	38 months (median)	81% (5 years) [salvage]—87% (5 years) [virgin]	/	/	94% (5 years) [salvage]—91% (5 years) [virgin]	/
Page C et al. (2013) [15]	291	T1-T3	56 months (mean)	80% (5 years)	/	/	/	93.94% (5 years)
Ozturk K et al. (2016) [5]	90	T1b—T2—selected T3	55 months (median)	80.4% (5 years)	/	76.7% (5 years)	/	/
Gong H et al. (2019) [16]	164	T1b—T2—selected T3	85 months (median)	86.9% (5 years)	87.6% (5 years)	82.4% (5 years)	/	/

Number of treated patients, stage of tumor (pT), period of follow up, overall survival (OS), disease-specific survival (DSS), disease-free survival (DFS), laryngeal preservation (LP), and local control (LC).

3.3. Salvage OPHL Type II

This group included five articles [10,11,19–21] (Table 2). Three studies [10,20,21] demonstrated that salvage OPHL type II guaranteed over 80% of 5-year overall survival. However, Deganello et al. [16] reported a 5-year OS of 60%. The 5-year LP was guaranteed in more than 90% of patients [10,19]: the use of total laryngectomy was, therefore, avoided in a really high percentage of patients. Pellini et al. [20] also reported excellent results in 5-year DFS (95.5%) in a sample of 70 patients; Bertolin et al. [21] obtained 86% of 5-year DFS in a sample of 50 patients.

Table 2. Salvage OPHL type II: characteristics of included studies.

Authors (Year of Publication)	N° Patients	pT Treated	Follow-Up	OS	DSS	DFS	LP	LC
Deganello A et al. (2008) [19]	31	T1-T4	45 months (mean)	60% (5 years)	/	/	90% (5 years)	75% (5 years)
Pellini R et al. (2008) [20]	78	T1-T4	70 months (median)	81.8% (5 years)	/	95.5% (5 years)	/	/
Nakayama M et al. (2013) [11]	30	T1-T4	38 months (median)	81% (5 years) [salvage]—87% (5 years) [primary]	/	/	94% (5 years) [salvage]—91% (5 years) [primary]	/
Sperry SM et al. (2013) [10]	42	T1-T3	61 months (mean)	75% (5 years)	85% (5 years)	/	95% (5 years)	98% (5 years)
Bertolin A et al. (2020) [21]	50	T1-T4	50.1 months (mean)	82% (5 years)	88% (5 years)	86% (5 years)	/	/

Number of treated patients, stage of tumor (pT), period of follow up, overall survival (OS), disease-specific survival (DSS), disease-free survival (DFS), laryngeal preservation (LP), and local control (LC).

3.4. Adjuvant Radiotherapy after Primary OPHL Type II

Eight articles assessed the oncological outcome of OPHL type II combined with adjuvant radiotherapy [8,13,22–27] (Table 3). Overall, adjuvant RT proved to be adequate for: positive resection margin, thyroid cartilage invasion (stage T4a), positive neck nodes with extracapsular invasion, multiple nodal metastases, following the National Comprehensive Cancer Network (NCCN) [28] guidelines. The majority of the studies reported 5-year OS and DSS higher than 80%. Rizzotto et al. [24] obtained 5-year OS and DFS in 95.6% and 90.9% of patients respectively. Basaran et al. [13] divided patients into two groups: (1) both arytenoids preserved (BASCL) and (2) one arytenoid preserved (OASCL). Overall, no statistically significant differences were detected in the two groups in terms of oncological outcome.

Table 3. Adjuvant radiotherapy after primary OPHL type II: characteristics of included studies.

Authors (Year of Publication)	N° Patients	pT Treated	Follow-Up	OS	DSS	DFS	LP	LC	LR	Criteria for Adjuvant RT
Gallo A et al. (2005) [20]	253	T1-T4	51.6 months (mean)	79.1% (5 years)	/	/	/	/	8.7% (5 years)	Positive resection margin, >N1, extracapsular spread
Pinar et al. (2012) [8]	56	T1-T4	58 months (median)	82.1% (5 years)	86.5% (5 years)	/	/	92.5% (5 years)	/	Positive resection margin, >N1, extracapsular spread, thyroid cartilage invasion
Topaloglu I et al. (2012) [23]	44	T2-T3	53.2 months (mean)	84.1% (5 years)	92.5% (5 years)	/	/	/	/	Positive resection margin, >N1, extracapsular spread, thyroid cartilage invasion
Rizzotto G et al. (2012) [24]	399	T1-T4	97 months (mean)	95.6% (5 years)	/	90.9% (5 years)	/	/	3.2% (5 years)	Positive resection margin, >N1, extracapsular spread
Mercante G et al. (2013) [25]	32	T3	47.3 months (median)	87.3% (5 years)	/	78.2% (5 years)	/	96.2% (5 years)	/	>N1, extracapsular spread, T4a
Basaran B et al. (2015) [13]	68	T2-T3	52.4 months (mean)	81.2% (5 years) [BASCL]—85% (5 years) [OASCL] p-value 0.66	93% (5 years) [BASCL]—89.5% (5 years) [OASCL] p-value 0.49	/	88.7% (5 years) [BASCL]—89.2% (5 years) [OASCL] p-value 0.59	86.8% (5 years) [BASCL]—84.2% (5 years) [OASCL] p-value 0.42	/	>N1, extracapsular spread
Atallah I et al. (2017) [26]	53	T1-T2	96 months (median)	93.7% (5 years)	95.6% (5 years)	87.7% (5 years)	/	/	11.3% (5 years)	Positive resection margin
Pescetto B et al. (2018) [27]	53	T1-T3	40.8 months (median)	86% (3 years)	95% (3 years)	80% (3 years)	/	/	/	/

Number of treated patients, stage of tumor (pT), period of follow up, overall survival (OS), disease-specific survival (DSS), disease-free survival (DFS), laryngeal preservation (LP), and local control (LC), local recurrence (LR), OASCL, both arytenoids preserved SCPL (BASCL), one arytenoid preserved SCPL (OASCL).

4. Discussion

Laryngeal carcinoma accounts for about 2% of all cancers in the world [29]. For early and locally advanced laryngeal cancers, several therapeutic strategies are available: TLM, radiotherapy, chemoradiotherapy and open laryngeal organ preservation surgery (OLOPS) [30–33].

In particular, supracricoid laryngectomy is an open partial laryngeal surgery that has two main goals: radical excision of laryngeal cancer and preservation of functions (swallowing, phonation and breathing). In fact, while removing portions of the larynx, this surgery, in its reconstructive phase, allows for restoring the physiological crossway between the digestive and respiratory tract.

OPHL type II is, therefore, recommended for selected supraglottic and glottic cancers [6], in which it manages to guarantee good oncological and functional outcomes, thus, limiting the use of both primary and salvage total laryngectomy. In particular, in 2018, the American Society of Clinical Oncology (ASCO) recommended: TLM or radiotherapy for T1 and T2 laryngeal cancers with the goal of preserving the larynx; OPHL or chemoradiotherapy for locally advanced disease (T3, T4 laryngeal cancers), in order to achieve the greatest possible organ preservation with minimal functional impairment; total laryngectomy for extensive T3 and T4a lesions for a better survival rate [4].

In regard to chemotherapy for locally advanced disease, in the same paper, ASCO stated that concurrent chemoradiotherapy (CRT) guarantees satisfactory results in terms of laryngeal preservation compared to RT alone, although with high in-field toxicity [4]. Furthermore, ASCO advised against induction chemotherapy before laryngeal preservation surgery, even though Luna-Ortiz et al. [34] proved that induction chemotherapy allowed one to perform OPHL type II even in the case of arytenoid fixation (which is a contraindication to this surgical technique) determining the recovery of motility, without any impairment of DFS and/or OS.

As for total laryngectomy, it represents a real amputation of an organ that strongly characterizes the individual and that is essential for breathing, swallowing and speaking. Furthermore, this surgery involves the creation of a permanent tracheostoma which creates an important and significant impact on the patient's psychology and overall quality of life [35]. Weinsten et al. [36] compared the quality of life using the SF-36 general health status system and the V-RQOL (Voice-Related Quality Of Life) test [37,38], showing significantly better results in the OPHL type II group compared to the total laryngectomy group.

However, patient selection is mandatory to provide the best treatment in both oncological and functional terms [9]. This selection is based not only on the characteristics of the tumor, i.e., localization and local-regional extension, but also on the health and psychosocial state of the patient himself. Therefore, from the oncologic point of view, OPHL type II is indicated in the case of T2 and selected T3 glottic and supraglottic cancers. The most important factors based on the patient's characteristics, on the other hand, are: age, intellectual abilities and pulmonary function [21]. In particular, the patient's age parameter (cut-off 70 years) [31] has always been the subject of discussion and debate. According to some authors, in fact, advanced age does not represent a contraindication to the intervention of OPHL type II [6] due to the difference between biological and chronological age [31]. According to other authors, however, advanced age correlates with a worse functional and clinical outcome [39]. Furthermore, Lucioni et al. [40] indicated young age as a negative prognostic factor, probably due to the increased aggressiveness of the tumor. Crosetti et al. identified other exclusion criteria: severe metabolic diseases, neurological and/or pulmonary diseases that compromise the ability to swallow and expectorate, severe heart diseases [41].

Finally, the choice of the best therapeutic strategy should always be agreed with the patient and with the family members too, highlighting the importance of involving the family in the final decision, making them aware of the therapeutic options and the advantages and disadvantages of each [10].

4.1. Primary OPHL Type II

Primary OPHL type II is recommended in cases of T2 and selected T3 glottic and supraglottic cancers. In particular, the American Society of Clinical Oncology suggests OPHL type II as first choice for T2 tumors because it achieves better oncological outcomes than primary RT [42]. ASCO also clarified that laryngeal preservation surgery should always be preferred to RT for T1 and T2 laryngeal cancer but underlined that TLM is not always feasible depending on these key points: endoscopic tumor exposure, endoscopic technique safety and surgeon's experience [4]. In fact, performing surgery with the awareness of not being radical (close or positive resection margins) and, therefore, of having to do post-operative RT, is not an acceptable therapeutic option in any way. For this reason, in these cases, OPHL type II represents a valid alternative to the TLM, before RT.

Moreover, surgery is preferred to RT because of toxicity, odynophagia, hoarseness and thick salivary secretions and, above all, it could relate to a high risk of dysphagia and aspiration. The selected articles showed the efficacy of primary OPHL type II as far as 5-year OS, DSS, DFS, LP, LC and LR are concerned. In their study, Page et al. [17] found some factors that relates to a statistically significant risk of local recurrence: age, lymph node positivity (N+), positive resection margin, other synchronous cancer. Furthermore, in their study, they underlined that the main risk factor for local recurrence (and, therefore, a negative prognostic factor) is the positive or close resection margins (healthy tissue-carcinoma distance <1 mm), especially the inferior margin [43]. For this reason, to guarantee a safe surgery, Page et al. stated that resection margins had to be superior to 1 mm and subglottic extension inferior to 10 mm.

4.2. Salvage OPHL Type II

Taking into consideration the choice and the clinical conditions of the patient, as well as the care center, selected glottic and supraglottic carcinomas can be treated with primary radiotherapy [19]. In fact, RT guarantees the preservation of laryngeal anatomical structures and, therefore, a better functional result. Furthermore, in some cases, a tracheostomy is not necessary and, consequently, has a lower impact on the patient's quality of life. However, this treatment has a recurrence rate between 5 and 30%, apart from the above-cited side effects. Atallah et al. found several factors that correlate to low local control rate in the case of RT for T2 glottic tumors: male sex, degree of tumor differentiation, administration modality of radiotherapy (total dose and fractionation of administration), the extension of the tumor to a subglottic level or the anterior commissure. In particular, in the latter case, the high risk of tumor recurrence or persistence is related to diagnostic and therapeutic limitations: (1) the difficulty of evaluating the possible involvement of the thyroid and cricoid cartilages and of the cricothyroid membrane and (2) the difficulty of irradiating this laryngeal region [26]. Thus, in these cases, OPHL type II is performed with two goals: safe tumor clearance and preservation of laryngeal functions [19]. However, it is important to underline that salvage surgery correlates to a high risk of complications (chondritis, salivary fistula, rupture of pexy) related to previous laryngeal irradiation. In fact, radiotherapy is responsible for a slow healing process with a delay in tracheal decannulation and recovery of swallowing function [44]. Nevertheless, the risk-benefit ratio in salvage OPHL type II is positive. Indeed, a valid disease local control emerged with OS, LP, and LC values being, on average, slightly lower than primary OPHL type II from the analysis of the selected articles. Furthermore, Pellini et al. [20] underlined that the recurrence after RT had a different diffusion pathway compared to virgin neoplasia, with tumor foci also being far from the initial site of the tumor. This concept still emphasizes the importance of a wide resection with safe surgical margins and frozen sections of the resection margins, although the evaluation is more problematic in tissues that have been previously radio-treated [11]. Nevertheless, in order to obtain satisfying oncological outcomes, the strict selection of the patients that can undergo partial laryngectomy is fundamental: therefore, it is not possible to consider OPHL type II as the standard salvage therapy [21].

4.3. Adjuvant Radiotherapy after Primary OPHL Type II

In different studies, OPHL type II was associated with adjuvant RT. As a consequence, in order to avoid bias on the results, these articles were assessed separately from those that calculated the oncological outcomes after surgery (OPHL type II). All the studies included in the review showed satisfying results, with 5-year OS, DSS, LP and LC superior to 85%, on average. These results confirm what was stated by Atallah et al. [26]: combined therapy (surgery and adjuvant RT) gives a better local control than surgery or radiotherapy alone.

However, if post-operative RT guarantees improved oncological results, on the other hand, the risk of significant impairment of the functions of the residual larynx increases [19].

4.4. The Old Discussion: Laryngeal Preservation vs. Functional Preservation

The Achilles' heel of OPHL, especially OPHL type II and type III, is the functional result in terms of voice and swallowing. In fact, these two functions are closely linked and interdependent: both depend on the ability of arytenoid(s) to perform the sphincter function. This depends more on the base of the tongue and the mucous thickness of neoglottis and arytenoids than on the motility and number of residual arytenoids or on the presence or absence of the epiglottis. Several studies have analyzed voice results in these patients and found a moderate to severe alteration in the quality of the voice [45]. However, as Schindler et al. stated, the voice, although qualitatively poor, is not perceived by the patient as a handicap characterizing the quality of life [46]. OPHL's functional success is assessed on the basis of two main parameters: decannulation and nasogastric feeding-tube (NFT) removal. In this respect, the literature data were highly variable: Pinar et al. [8] reported a mean nasogastric tube removal of 11.43 days and a decannulation time of 16.79 days, On the contrary, Goncalves et al. [47] removed NFT and tracheal tube with a mean of 69 and 60 days, respectively. However, the decannulation rates were very high (over 85%), confirming good neoglottic patency [8,48]. In the case of impaired neoglottic patency, especially in patients with a poor cough reflex, tracheal aspiration (not only during feeding but constantly with saliva) can cause a serious complication, that is, aspiration pneumonia, with a lower than 20% incidence [47]. In the most serious cases, with frequent episodes of aspiration pneumonia, it is necessary to resort to total laryngectomy for a dysfunctional larynx with a very low rate (less than 2%) [49]. In fact, unfortunately, the preservation of the organ does not always correspond to function preservation, both in the case of surgery and RT. Therefore, in the choice of the best therapeutic approach for the patient with laryngeal carcinoma, it is mandatory to consider pros and cons of therapy and to determine, together with the patient, the best therapeutic strategy in terms of both oncology and function.

4.5. Study Limitation

First of all, despite the use of strict selection criteria, the included articles were heterogeneous in terms of number of patients and stage of larynx carcinoma. Indeed, it was impossible to analyze the oncological outcome considering the larynx carcinoma because the selected articles showed an overall result over the total number of treated patients. Furthermore, differentiating the oncological outcomes between OPHL type IIa and IIb was impossible in the review, because very few studies showed diversified results for these two categories.

5. Conclusions

The systematic analysis of the articles demonstrated that OPHL type II is useful to obtain oncological radicality. Indeed, this surgical technique proved to be efficient both as primary and salvage surgery. Furthermore, the study showed another important element: the strict selection of patients eligible for OPHL, based not only on the tumor's characteristics but also on the health and psychosocial conditions of the patient himself.

6. Highlights

- OPHL type II has two aims: oncological radicality and organ preservation
- OPHL type II ensures good oncological outcome both in primary and salvage surgery
- OPHL type II performs better results in primary surgery than in salvage surgery
- The main criterion for positive outcomes is the strict selection of patient and tumor stage

Author Contributions: Conceptualization, C.S.; methodology, C.S.; validation, C.S., F.G.; formal analysis, F.G.; investigation, B.V.; resources, B.V.; data curation, B.V., F.C.; writing—original draft preparation, C.S.; writing—review and editing, C.S., F.C.; supervision, C.S., F.G. All authors have read and agreed to the published version of the manuscript.

Funding: This research received no external funding.

Institutional Review Board Statement: Not applicable.

Informed Consent Statement: Not applicable.

Data Availability Statement: Publicly available datasets were analyzed in this study. This data can be found here: https://pubmed.ncbi.nlm.nih.gov/, accessed on 30 January 2021.

Conflicts of Interest: The authors declare no conflict of interest.

References

1. Majer, E.H.; Rieder, W. Technic of laryngectomy permitting the conservation of respiratory permeability (cricohyoidopexy). *Les Ann. D'oto-Laryngol.* **1959**, *76*, 677–681.
2. Piquet, J.J.; Desaulty, A.; Decroix, G. La crico-hyoïdo-épiglotto-pexie. Technique opératoire et résultats fonctionnels. *Ann. Otolaryngol. Chir. Cervicofac.* **1974**, *91*, 681–686. [PubMed]
3. Karasalihoglu, A.R.; Yagiz, R.; Tas, A.; Uzun, C.; Adali, M.K.; Koten, M. Supracricoid partial laryngectomy with cricohyoidopexy and cricohyoidoepiglottopexy: Functional and oncological results. *J. Laryngol. Otol.* **2004**, *118*, 671–675. [CrossRef] [PubMed]
4. Forastiere, A.A.; Ismaila, N.; Lewin, J.; Nathan, C.A.; Adelstein, D.J.; Eisbruch, A.; Fass, G.; Fisher, S.G.; Laurie, S.A.; Le, Q.-T.; et al. Use of Larynx-Preservation Strategies in the Treatment of Laryngeal Cancer: American Society of Clinical Oncology Clinical Practice Guideline Update. *J. Clin. Oncol.* **2018**, *36*, 1143–1169. [CrossRef] [PubMed]
5. Ozturk, K.; Akyildiz, S.; Gode, S.; Turhal, G.; Kirazli, T.; Aysel, A.; Uluoz, U. Post-Surgical and Oncologic Outcomes of Supracricoid Partial Laryngectomy: A Single-Institution Report of Ninety Cases. *ORL J. Otorhinolaryngol. Relat. Spec.* **2016**, *78*, 86–93. [CrossRef] [PubMed]
6. Sánchez-Cuadrado, I.; Castro, A.; Bernáldez, R.; Del Palacio, A.; Gavilán, J. Oncologic Outcomes after Supracricoid Partial Laryngectomy. *Otolaryngol. Head Neck Surg.* **2011**, *144*, 910–914. [CrossRef] [PubMed]
7. Succo, G.; Peretti, G.; Piazza, C.; Remacle, M.; Eckel, H.E.; Chevalier, D.; Simo, R.; Hantzakos, A.G.; Rizzotto, G.; Lucioni, M.; et al. Open partial horizontal laryngectomies: A proposal for classification by the working committee on nomenclature of the European Laryngological Society. *Eur. Arch. Oto-Rhino-Laryngol.* **2014**, *271*, 2489–2496. [CrossRef]
8. Pinar, E.; Imre, A.; Calli, C.; Oncel, S.; Katilmis, H. Supracricoid Partial Laryngectomy: Analyses of oncologic and functional outcomes. *Otolaryngol. Head Neck Surg.* **2012**, *147*, 1093–1098. [CrossRef] [PubMed]
9. Calearo, C.; Bignardi, L. A personal experience with subtotal and conservation surgery as treatment for laryngeal cancer. *Eur. Arch. Oto-Rhino-Laryngol.* **1986**, *243*, 174–179. [CrossRef]
10. Sperry, S.M.; Rassekh, C.H.; Laccourreye, O.; Weinstein, G.S. Supracricoid Partial Laryngectomy for Primary and Recurrent Laryngeal Cancer. *JAMA Otolaryngol. Head Neck Surg.* **2013**, *139*, 1226–1235. [CrossRef]
11. Nakayama, M.; Okamoto, M.; Hayakawa, K.; Ishiyama, H.; Kotani, S.; Miyamoto, S.; Seino, Y.; Okamoto, T.; Soda, I.; Sekiguchi, A. Clinical outcome of supracricoid laryngectomy with cricohyoidoepiglottopexy: Radiation failure versus previously untreated patients. *Auris Nasus Larynx* **2013**, *40*, 207–210. [CrossRef]
12. Cho, K.J.; Joo, Y.H.; Sun, D.I.; Kim, M.S. Supracricoid laryngectomy: Oncologic validity and functional safety. *Eur. Arch. Oto-Rhino-Laryngol.* **2010**, *267*, 1919–1925. [CrossRef]
13. Basaran, B.; Ünsaler, S.; Ulusan, M.; Aslan, I. The Effect of Arytenoidectomy on Functional and Oncologic Results of Supracricoid Partial Laryngectomy. *Ann. Otol. Rhinol. Laryngol.* **2015**, *124*, 788–796. [CrossRef] [PubMed]
14. Mattioli, F.; Fermi, M.; Molinari, G.; Capriotti, V.; Melegari, G.; Bertolini, F.; D'Angelo, E.; Tirelli, G.; Presutti, L. pT3 N0 Laryngeal Squamous Cell Carcinoma: Oncologic Outcomes and Prognostic Factors of Surgically Treated Patients. *Laryngoscope* **2021**, *131*, 2262–2268. [CrossRef] [PubMed]
15. Crosetti, E.; Bertolin, A.; Molteni, G.; Bertotto, I.; Balmativola, D.; Carraro, M.; Sprio, A.E.; Berta, G.N.; Presutti, L.; Rizzotto, G.; et al. Patterns of recurrence after open partial horizontal laryngectomy types II and III: Univariate and logistic regression analysis of risk factors. *Acta Otorhinolaryngol. Ital.* **2019**, *39*, 235–243. [CrossRef] [PubMed]

16. Moher, D.; Liberati, A.; Tetzlaff, J.; Altman, D.G.; PRISMA Group. Preferred reporting items for systematic reviews and meta-analyses: The PRISMA statement. *PLoS Med.* **2009**, *6*, e1000097. [CrossRef]
17. Page, C.; Mortuaire, G.; Mouawad, F.; Ganry, O.; Darras, J.; Pasquesoone, X.; Chevalier, D. Supracricoid laryngectomy with cricohyoidoepiglottopexy (CHEP) in the management of laryngeal carcinoma: Oncologic results. A 35-year experience. *Eur. Arch. Oto-Rhino-Laryngol.* **2013**, *270*, 1927–1932. [CrossRef]
18. Gong, H.; Zhou, L.; Wu, H.; Tao, L.; Chen, X.; Li, X.; Li, C.; Zhou, J. Long-term clinical outcomes of supracricoid partial laryngectomy with cricohyoidoepiglottopexy for glottic carcinoma. *Acta Oto-Laryngol.* **2019**, *139*, 803–809. [CrossRef] [PubMed]
19. Deganello, A.; Gallo, O.; De Cesare, J.M.; Ninu, M.B.; Gitti, G.; Campora, L.D.; Radici, M.; Campora, E.D. Supracricoid partial laryngectomy as salvage surgery for radiation therapy failure. *Head Neck* **2008**, *30*, 1064–1071. [CrossRef]
20. Pellini, R.; Pichi, B.; Ruscito, P.; Ceroni, A.R.; Caliceti, U.; Rizzotto, G.; Pazzaia, A.; Laudadio, P.; Piazza, C.; Peretti, G.; et al. Supracricoid partial laryngectomies after radiation failure: A multi-institutional series. *Head Neck* **2008**, *30*, 372–379. [CrossRef]
21. Bertolin, A.; Lionello, M.; Ghizzo, M.; Cena, I.; Leone, F.; Valerini, S.; Mattioli, F.; Crosetti, E.; Presutti, L.; Succo, G.; et al. Salvage open partial horizontal laryngectomy after failed radiotherapy: A multicentric study. *Laryngoscope* **2020**, *130*, 431–436. [CrossRef]
22. Gallo, A.; Manciocco, V.; Simonelli, M.; Pagliuca, G.; D'Arcangelo, E.; de Vincentiis, M. Supracricoid Partial Laryngectomy in the Treatment of Laryngeal Cancer: UnIn Proceedings of theivariate and multivariate analysis of prognostic factors. *Arch. Otolaryngol.—Head Neck Surg.* **2005**, *131*, 620–625. [CrossRef] [PubMed]
23. Topaloğlu, I.; Bal, M.; Saltürk, Z. Supracricoid laryngectomy with cricohyoidopexy: Oncological results. *Eur. Arch. Oto-Rhino-Laryngol.* **2011**, *269*, 1959–1965. [CrossRef]
24. Rizzotto, G.; Crosetti, E.; Lucioni, M.; Succo, G. Subtotal laryngectomy: Outcomes of 469 patients and proposal of a comprehensive and simplified classification of surgical procedures. *Eur. Arch. Oto-Rhino-Laryngol.* **2012**, *269*, 1635–1646. [CrossRef]
25. Mercante, G.; Grammatica, A.; Battaglia, P.; Cristalli, G.; Pellini, R.; Spriano, G. Supracricoid Partial Laryngectomy in the Management of T3 Laryngeal Cancer. *Otolaryngol. Head Neck Surg.* **2013**, *149*, 714–720. [CrossRef] [PubMed]
26. Atallah, I.; Berta, E.; Coffre, A.; Villa, J.; Reyt, E.; Righini, C. Supracricoid partial laryngectomy with crico-hyoido-epiglottopexy for glottic carcinoma with anterior commissure involvement. La laringectomia parziale sopracricoidea con crico-ioido-pessia per il carcinoma della glottide coinvolgente la commissura anteriore. *Acta Otorhinolaryngol. Ital.* **2017**, *37*, 188–194. [CrossRef]
27. Pescetto, B.; Gal, J.; Chamorey, E.; Dassonville, O.; Poissonnet, G.; Bozec, A. Role of supracricoid partial laryngectomy with cricohyoidoepiglottopexy in glottic carcinoma with anterior commissure involvement. *Eur. Ann. Otorhinolaryngol. Head Neck Dis.* **2018**, *135*, 249–253. [CrossRef]
28. Pfister, D.G.; Spencer, S.; Adelstein, D.; Adkins, D.; Anzai, Y.; Brizel, D.M.; Bruce, J.Y.; Busse, P.M.; Caudell, J.J.; Cmelak, A.J.; et al. Head and Neck Cancers, Version 2.2020, NCCN Clinical Practice Guidelines in Oncology. *J. Natl. Compr. Cancer Netw.* **2020**, *18*, 873–898. [CrossRef] [PubMed]
29. Succo, G.; Crosetti, E.; Bertolin, A.; Lucioni, M.; Caracciolo, A.; Panetta, V.; Sprio, A.E.; Berta, G.N.; Rizzotto, G. Benefits and drawbacks of open partial horizontal laryngectomies, Part A: Early- to intermediate-stage glottic carcinoma. *Head Neck* **2016**, *38* (Suppl. S1), E333–E340. [CrossRef]
30. Vella, O.; Blanchard, D.; de Raucourt, D.; Rame, J.E.; Babin, E. Function evaluation of laryngeal reconstruction using infrahyoid muscle after partial laryngectomy in 37 patients. *Eur. Ann. Otorhinolaryngol. Head Neck Dis.* **2020**, *137*, 7–11. [CrossRef]
31. Succo, G.; Crosetti, E. Limitations and Opportunities in Open Laryngeal Organ Preservation Surgery: Current Role of OPHLs. *Front. Oncol.* **2019**, *9*, 408. [CrossRef]
32. Nguyen, N.P.; Chi, A.; Betz, M.; Almeida, F.; Vos, P.; Davis, R.; Slane, B.; Ceizyk, M.; Abraham, D.; Smith-Raymond, L.; et al. Feasibility of Intensity-Modulated and Image-Guided Radiotherapy for Functional Organ Preservation in Locally Advanced Laryngeal Cancer. *PLoS ONE* **2012**, *7*, e42729. [CrossRef]
33. Kim, K.N.; Dyer, M.A.; Qureshi, M.M.; Shah, N.K.; Grillone, G.A.; Faden, D.L.; Jalisi, S.M.; Truong, M.T. Hypofractionated radiotherapy and surgery compared to standard radiotherapy in early glottic cancer. *Am. J. Otolaryngol.* **2020**, *41*, 102544. [CrossRef]
34. Luna-Ortiz, K.; Reynoso-Noveron, N.; Zacarias-Ramon, L.C.; Alvarez-Avitia, M.; Luna-Peteuil, Z.; Garcia-Ortega, D.Y. Supracricoid Partial Laryngectomy With and Without Neoadjuvant Chemotherapy in Glottic Cancer. *Laryngoscope* **2021**, *132*, 156–162. [CrossRef] [PubMed]
35. Massaro, N.; Verro, B.; Greco, G.; Chianetta, E.; D'Ecclesia, A.; Saraniti, C. Quality of Life with Voice Prosthesis after Total Laryngectomy. *Iran J. Otorhinolaryngol.* **2021**, *33*, 301–309. [CrossRef] [PubMed]
36. Weinstein, G.S.; El-Sawy, M.M.; Ruiz, C.; Dooley, P.; Chalian, A.; El-Sayed, M.M.; Goldberg, A. Laryngeal Preservation With Supracricoid Partial Laryngectomy Results in Improved Quality of Life When Compared With Total Laryngectomy. *Laryngoscope* **2001**, *111*, 191–199. [CrossRef]
37. Ware, J.E.; Kosinski, M.; Keller, S.D. *SF-36 Physical and Mental Health Summary Scale: A User Manual*; The Health Institute, New England Medical Center: Boston, UK, 1994.
38. Hogikyan, N.D.; Sethuraman, G. Validation of an instrument to measure voice-related quality of life (V-RQOL). *J. Voice* **1999**, *13*, 557–569. [CrossRef]
39. Fantini, M.; Crosetti, E.; Affaniti, R.; Sprio, A.E.; Bertotto, I.; Succo, G. Preoperative prognostic factors for functional and clinical outcomes after open partial horizontal laryngectomies. *Head Neck* **2021**, *43*, 3459–3467. [CrossRef]

40. Lucioni, M.; Bertolin, A.; Lionello, M.; Giacomelli, L.; Rizzotto, G.; Marioni, G. Salvage transoral laser microsurgery for recurrent glottic carcinoma after primary laser-assisted treatment: Analysis of prognostic factors. *Head Neck* **2016**, *38*, 1043–1049. [CrossRef]
41. Crosetti, E.; Caracciolo, A.; Molteni, G.; Sprio, A.E.; Berta, G.; Presutti, L. Unravelling the risk factors that underlie laryngeal surgery in elderly, Svelare i fattori di rischio che sottendono la chirurgia laringea negli anziani. *Acta Otorhinolaryngol. Ital.* **2016**, *36*, 185–193. [CrossRef]
42. American Society of Clinical Oncology; Pfister, D.G.; Laurie, S.A.; Weinstein, G.S.; Mendenhall, W.M.; Adelstein, D.J.; Ang, K.K.; Clayman, G.L.; Fisher, S.G.; Forastiere, A.A.; et al. American Society of Clinical Oncology Clinical Practice Guideline for the Use of Larynx-Preservation Strategies in the Treatment of Laryngeal Cancer. *J. Clin. Oncol.* **2006**, *24*, 3693–3704. [CrossRef]
43. Saraniti, C.; Montana, F.; Chianetta, E.; Greco, G.; Verro, B. Impact of resection margin status and revision transoral laser microsurgery in early glottic cancer: Analysis of organ preservation and disease local control on a cohort of 153 patients. *Braz. J. Otorhinolaryngol.* **2020**, 1808. [CrossRef] [PubMed]
44. Makeieff, M.; Venegoni, D.; Mercante, G.; Crampette, L.; Guerrier, B. Supracricoid Partial Laryngectomies after Failure of Radiation Therapy. *Laryngoscope* **2005**, *115*, 353–357. [CrossRef] [PubMed]
45. Schindler, A.; Pizzorni, N.; Mozzanica, F.; Fantini, M.; Ginocchio, D.; Bertolin, A.; Crosetti, E.; Succo, G. Functional outcomes after supracricoid laryngectomy: What do we not know and what do we need to know? *Eur. Arch. Oto-Rhino-Laryngol.* **2015**, *273*, 3459–3475. [CrossRef]
46. Schindler, A.; Mozzanica, F.; Ginocchio, D.; Invernizzi, A.; Peri, A.; Ottaviani, F. Voice-related quality of life in patients after total and partial laryngectomy. *Auris Nasus Larynx* **2012**, *39*, 77–83. [CrossRef] [PubMed]
47. Gonçalves, A.; Bertelli, A.; Malavasi, T.; Kikuchi, W.; Rodrigues, A.; Menezes, M. Results after supracricoid horizontal partial laryngectomy. *Auris Nasus Larynx* **2010**, *37*, 84–88. [CrossRef]
48. Saraniti, C.; Speciale, R.; Santangelo, M.; Massaro, N.; Maniaci, A.; Gallina, S. Functional outcomes after supracricoid modified partial laryngectomy. *J. Biol. Regul. Homeost. Agents* **2019**, *33*, 1903–1907.
49. Thomas, L.; Drinnan, M.; Natesh, B.; Mehanna, H.; Jones, T.; Paleri, V. Open conservation partial laryngectomy for laryngeal cancer: A systematic review of English language literature. *Cancer Treat. Rev.* **2012**, *38*, 203–211. [CrossRef]

Article

Increased Risk of Neurodegenerative Dementia after Benign Paroxysmal Positional Vertigo

So Young Kim [1], Dae Myoung Yoo [2], Chanyang Min [2,3] and Hyo Geun Choi [2,4,*]

1. Department of Otorhinolaryngology-Head & Neck Surgery, CHA Bundang Medical Center, CHA University, Seongnam 13496, Korea; sossi81@hanmail.net
2. Hallym Data Science Laboratory, Hallym University, College of Medicine, Anyang 14068, Korea; ydm1285@naver.com (D.M.Y.); joicemin@naver.com (C.M.)
3. Graduate School of Public Health, Seoul National University, Seoul 08826, Korea
4. Department of Otorhinolaryngology-Head & Neck Surgery, Hallym University College of Medicine, Anyang 14068, Korea
* Correspondence: pupen@naver.com

Abstract: The aim of the present study was to estimate the risk of dementia in patients with benign paroxysmal positional vertigo (BPPV), using a population cohort. Data from the Korean National Health Insurance Service-National Sample Cohort for the population ≥60 years of age from 2002 to 2013 were collected. A total of 11,432 individuals with dementia were matched for age, sex, income, region of residence, hypertension, diabetes, and dyslipidemia with 45,728 individuals comprising the control group. The crude (simple) and adjusted odds ratios (ORs) of dementia in BPPV patients were analyzed using non-conditional logistic regression analyses. Subgroup analyses were conducted according to age and sex. A history of BPPV characterized 5.3% (609/11,432) of the dementia group and 2.6% (1,194/45,728) of the control group ($p < 0.001$). The adjusted OR of dementia for BPPV was 1.14 (95% CI = 1.03–1.26, $p = 0.009$). In subgroup analyses according to age and sex, males had higher ORs of dementia for BPPV. BPPV increases the risk of dementia in the 60 years of age or older population.

Keywords: benign paroxysmal positional vertigo; dementia; risk factors; cohort studies; epidemiology

1. Introduction

A cross-sectional study reported that patients with cognitive impairment, such as mild cognitive impairment and Alzheimer's dementia, show a high risk of vestibular dysfunction [1]. The vestibular system is known to affect cognitive functions, such as visuospatial ability, memory, and attention [2,3]. In a cross-sectional study that included 308 adults with neurodegenerative disorders, the authors observed that attentional and visuospatial cognitive abilities were correlated with increased dizziness [2]. Additionally, the prevalence of hippocampal atrophy was higher in patients with chronic bilateral vestibular dysfunction than in controls [4]. The authors hypothesized that optimal vestibular function is essential to maintain the phylogenetically ancient hippocampal function, such as spatial aspects of memory processing for navigation [5]. At the molecular level, unilateral vestibulopathy was associated with decreased hippocampal expression of N-methyl-D-aspartate receptors [4]. Therefore, it is reasonable to conclude that vestibular disorders may be associated with dementia.

Benign paroxysmal positional vertigo (BPPV) is the most common cause of vestibular vertigo in elderly individuals [6]; approximately 30% of individuals aged ≥70 years report an episode of BPPV at least once in their lifetime [7,8]. Moreover, the response to canalith repositioning therapy tends to be lower and the rate of recurrent BPPV is higher in elderly patients than in younger individuals [6,9,10]. BPPV shows a benign course; therefore, its association with other diseases is often ignored. A recent study reported BPPV as a predictor of dementia [11].

Both direct and indirect mechanisms may underlie the association between BPPV and dementia. With regard to a direct mechanism, an increased risk of falls in patients with BPPV may result in a high risk of head trauma and physical inactivity, which predispose these patients to dementia [1,12]. The sudden onset of vertigo observed in patients with BPPV reportedly increases the risk of falls in elderly patients [13]. With regard to indirect mechanisms, common cardiovascular or cerebrovascular pathophysiologies may mediate the onset of dementia in patients with BPPV. Recent studies have suggested a causal association between cardiovascular diseases, including hypertension and ischemic heart disease, and BPPV [14,15]. Vascular disorders, including hypertension, diabetes, and dyslipidemia, are known to increase the risk of dementia [16–18].

We hypothesized that BPPV could increase the risk of dementia. We searched the PubMed and Embase databases using the key words "BPPV" and "dementia" and included all entries until September 2021 in our search. We identified only one population cohort study that reported an increased risk of dementia in patients with BPPV [11]. However, the study did not include a control group matched for comorbidities. The characteristics of early-onset dementia differ from those of late-onset dementia; therefore, inclusion of individuals aged $\geq$20 years in a study with a follow-up of 10 years may negatively affect the association between dementia and BPPV [19]. In this study, we investigated the association between BPPV and dementia in an older Korean population extracted from a national sample cohort. This study extended previous research in the field; we investigated a history of BPPV as an independent risk factor in patients aged $\geq$60 years diagnosed with dementia.

2. Materials and Methods

2.1. Ethical Considerations

The Ethics Committee of Hallym University (2014-I148) approved the use of the data. The need for written informed consent was waived by the Institutional Review Board.

2.2. Study Population and Data Collection

This matched case–control study relied on data from the Korean National Health Insurance Service-National Sample Cohort (NHIS-NSC). The Korean NHIS selects samples directly from the database of the entire population to prevent non-sampling errors [20]. For this study, ~2% of the samples (one million) were selected from the entire Korean population (50 million). The selected data could be classified at 1476 levels (including age (18 categories), sex (2 categories), and income level (41 categories)) using randomized stratified systematic sampling methods via proportional allocation to represent the entire population. After data selection, the appropriateness of the sample was verified as described previously [21]. The details of the methods used to perform these procedures are provided by the National Health Insurance Sharing Service [22]. The cohort database used in our study included (i) personal information, (ii) health-insurance claim codes (procedures and prescriptions), (iii) diagnostic codes using the International Classification of Disease-10 (ICD-10), (iv) death records from the Korean National Statistical Office (using the Korean Standard Classification of disease), (v) socio-economic data (residence and income), and (vi) medical examination data for each participant during the period 2002–2013.

As all Korean citizens are assigned a 13-digit resident registration number that is retained from birth to death, exact population statistics can be determined from the resulting database. All Koreans must enroll in the NHIS. The 13-digit resident registration number is used by Korean hospitals and clinics to register individual patients in the medical insurance system. Therefore, the risk of overlapping medical records is minimal, even if a patient moves from one place to another. Moreover, all medical treatments in Korea can be tracked, without exception, using the HIRA (Health Insurance Review & Assessment Service) system. In Korea, a notice of death must be submitted to an administrative entity before a funeral can be held. The cause and date of death are recorded in the death certificate, which is prepared by a medical doctor.

2.3. Participant Selection

Among the 1,125,691 individuals with 114,369,638 medical claim codes, those diagnosed with dementia were included in the study. Dementia was defined based on a diagnosis of Alzheimer's disease (G30) or dementia in Alzheimer's disease (F00). To ensure the accuracy of the diagnosis, only those participants treated at least twice were included in the study. The reliability of the dementia diagnosis is described in the Supplemental Digital Content.

The study population consisted of 13,102 dementia patients diagnosed between 2002 and 2013. BPPV was diagnosed based on ICD-10 codes (H811) and at least two treatments for this condition between 2002 and 2013.

The dementia patients were matched 1:4 with members of a control group selected from the original population (n = 1,112,589) and consisting of individuals never diagnosed with dementia between 2002 and 2013. The matches were processed for age, sex, income, region of residence, and a medical history of hypertension, diabetes, or dyslipidemia. To prevent bias in the selection of matched participants, control-group participants were sorted by first assigning them a random number, which was then used in their selection, beginning with the highest and ending with the lowest number. It was assumed that the relation to the index date of the matched control participants was the same as that of each matched participant with dementia. Therefore, a person in the control group who died before the index date was excluded. Dementia participants for whom a sufficient number of matching control participants could not be identified were excluded (n = 1158), as were participants younger than 60 years of age who had been previously diagnosed with dementia (n = 514). In the young population, dementia is rare and often has a specific underlying etiology. Finally, using 1:4 matching, 11,432 dementia patients and 45,728 controls were included in the study (Figure 1). However, the two groups were not matched for ischemic heart disease and cerebral stroke history, as the stricter matching would have increased the exclusion of dementia patients due to a lack of controls. After matching, both groups were analyzed for a previous history of BPPV.

2.4. Variables

All variables including age, income level, region of residence, and comorbidities were based on the index date. Six age groups were defined according to 5-year intervals, ranging from 60–64 to 85+ years of age. Income groups were initially divided into 41 classes (1 health-insurance-assistance class, 20 self-employment health-insurance classes, and 20 employment health-insurance classes) but then re-categorized into five classes, ranging from lowest (class 1) to highest (class 5). Sixteen regions of residence were defined according to administrative district. These regions were regrouped as urban (Seoul, Busan, Daegu, Incheon, Gwangju, Daejeon, and Ulsan) and rural (Gyeonggi, Gangwon, Chungcheongbuk, Chungcheongnam, Jeollabuk, Jeollanam, Gyeongsangbuk, Gyeongsangnam, and Jeju).

The prior medical histories of the patients and controls were evaluated using ICD-10 codes. To ensure the accuracy of the diagnoses, hypertension (I10 and I15), diabetes (E10–E14), dyslipidemia (E78), and head trauma (S00–S09) were regarded as present if treated at least twice, and Meniere's disease (H810), ischemic heart disease (I24 and I25), and cerebral stroke (I60–I63) strokes as present if treated at least once.

2.5. Statistical Analyses

Chi-square tests were used to compare the general characteristics of the dementia and control groups. The odds ratio (ORs) of BPPV for dementia was analyzed using unconditional logistic regression analysis together with crude (simple) and adjusted (ischemic heart disease, stroke, Meniere's disease, and head-trauma histories) models and calculating 95% confidence intervals (CIs). Age, sex, income, region of residence, hypertension, diabetes mellitus, and dyslipidemia were stratified in a conditional logistic regression model. For the subgroup analyses, participants were divided with respect to age (<75 years old, ≥75 years), sex, income, region of residence, hypertension, diabetes, dyslipidemia, ischemic heart disease, stroke, Meniere's disease, and head trauma. Two-tailed analyses were conducted. A p value < 0.05 was considered to indicate statistical significance. The analyses were conducted using SPSS v. 22.0 (IBM, Armonk, NY, USA).

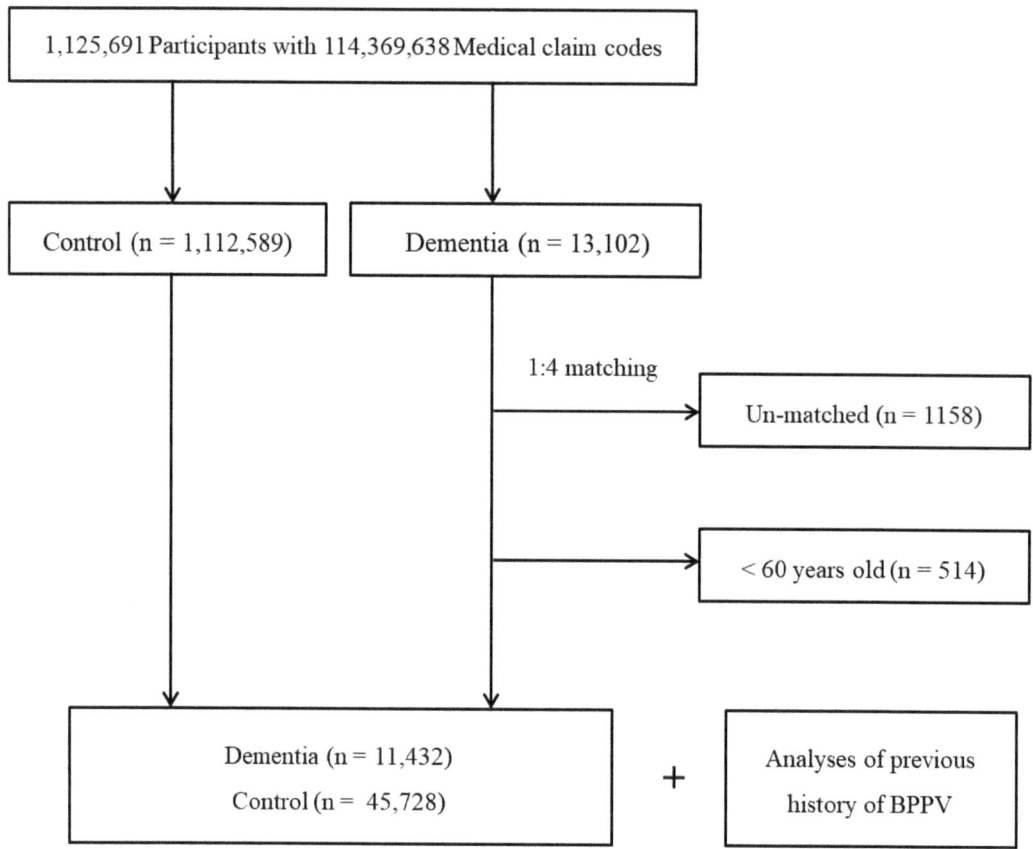

Figure 1. Schematic illustration of the participant-selection process used in the study. From a total of 1,125,691 participants, 11,432 patients with dementia were matched with 45,728 controls for age, sex, income, region of residence, and medical histories.

3. Results

A history of BPPV was documented in 5.3% (609/11,432) of the dementia patients vs. 2.6% of the controls (1194/45,728; $p < 0.001$, Table 1). The mean follow-up duration from BPPV to index date was 49.97 (standard deviation [SD] = 35.97) for the dementia group and 50.34 (SD = 33.90) for the control group. Age, sex, income, region of residence, and history of hypertension, diabetes, and dyslipidemia were matched between the dementia and control groups. A history of ischemic heart disease, cerebral stroke, Meniere's disease, and head trauma were higher in the dementia group than in the control group.

Table 1. General Characteristics of Participants.

Characteristics	Total Participants		
	Dementia (n, %)	Control Group (n, %)	Standardized Differences
Age (years old)			0.00
60–64	580 (5.1)	2320 (5.1)	
65–69	1289 (11.3)	5156 (11.3)	
70–74	2325 (20.3)	9300 (20.3)	
75–79	2978 (26.1)	11,912 (26.1)	
80–84	2705 (23.7)	10,820 (23.7)	
85+	1555 (13.6)	6220 (13.6)	
Sex			0.00
Male	3659 (32.0)	14,636 (32.0)	
Female	7773 (68.0)	31,092 (68.0)	
Income			
1 (lowest)	2858 (25.0)	11,432 (25.0)	0.00
2	1037 (9.1)	4148 (9.1)	
3	1371 (12.0)	5484 (12.0)	
4	1886 (16.5)	7544 (16.5)	
5 (highest)	4280 (37.4)	17,120 (37.4)	
Region of residence			0.00
Urban	4617 (40.4)	18,468 (40.4)	
Rural	6815 (59.6)	27,260 (59.6)	
Hypertension			0.00
Yes	8314 (72.7)	33,256 (72.7)	
No	3118 (27.3)	12,472 (27.3)	
Diabetes Mellitus			0.00
Yes	4060 (35.5)	16,240 (35.5)	
No	7372 (64.5)	29488 (64.5)	
Dyslipidemia			0.00
Yes	3558 (31.1)	14,232 (31.1)	
No	7874 (68.9)	31,496 (68.9)	
Ischemic heart disease			0.05
Yes	1703 (15.0)	5992 (13.1)	
No	9729 (85.1)	39,736 (86.9)	
Cerebral stroke			0.50
Yes	5524 (48.3)	11,475 (25.1)	
No	5908 (51.7)	34,253 (74.9)	
Meniere's disease			0.03
Yes	651 (5.7)	2319 (5.1)	
No	10,781 (94.3)	43,409 (94.9)	
Head trauma			0.03
Yes	886 (7.8)	1887 (4.1)	
No	10,546 (92.3)	43,841 (95.9)	
BPPV (Benging Paroxysmal Positional Vertigo)			0.05
Yes	609 (5.3)	1914 (2.6)	
No	10,823 (94.7)	43,814 (95.8)	

The OR for BPPV was higher in the dementia group than in the control group (OR = 1.29, 95% CI = 1.18–1.42; $p < 0.001$, Table 2). The higher risk was maintained after adjusting for ischemic heart disease, cerebral stroke, Meniere's disease, and head trauma (adjusted OR = 1.14, 95% CI = 1.03–1.26; $p = 0.009$).

Table 2. Crude and adjusted odds ratios (95% confidence interval) of BPPV for dementia and in subgroup analysis according to age, sex, income, and region of residence.

Characteristics	No. of BPPV/ No. of Dementia (%)	No. of BPPV/ No. of Control (%)	Crude†	p-Value	Adjusted †,‡	p-Value	p for Interaction
Total participants (n = 57,160)							
BPPV	609/11,432 (5.3)	1914/45,728 (4.2)	1.29 (1.18–1.42)	<0.001 *	1.14 (1.03–1.26)	0.009 *	
Age < 75 years old (n = 20,970)							
BPPV	216/4194 (5.2)	624/16,776 (3.7)	1.41 (1.20–1.65)	<0.001 *	1.18 (0.99–1.39)	0.062	0.245
Age ≥ 75 years old (n = 36,190)							
BPPV	393/7238 (5.4)	1290/28,952 (4.5)	1.23 (1.10–1.39)	<0.001 *	1.12 (0.99–1.26)	0.066	
Men (n = 18,295)							
BPPV	158/3659 (4.3)	428/14,636 (2.9)	1.50 (1.25–1.81)	<0.001 *	1.32 (1.09–1.61)	0.005 *	0.063
Women (n = 38,865)							
BPPV	451/7773 (5.8)	1486/31,092 (4.8)	1.23 (1.10–1.37)	<0.001 *	1.09 (0.97–1.22)	0.148	
Low income (n = 26,330)							
BPPV	262/5266 (5.0)	795/21,064 (3.8)	1.34 (1.16–1.55)	<0.001 *	1.19 (1.02–1.38)	0.026 *	0.651
High income (n = 30,830)							
BPPV	347/6166 (5.6)	1119/24,664 (4.5)	1.26 (1.11–1.42)	<0.001 *	1.10 (0.97–1.26)	0.134	
Urban (n = 23,085)							
BPPV	242/4617 (5.2)	762/18,468 (4.1)	1.29 (1.11–1.50)	0.001 *	1.14 (0.98–1.33)	0.096	0.920
Rural (n = 34,075)							
BPPV	367/6815 (5.4)	1152/27,260 (4.2)	1.29 (1.15–1.46)	<0.001 *	1.14 (1.00–1.29)	0.046 *	

* Odd ratios on unconditional logistic regression model, Significance at $p < 0.05$. † Age, sex, income, region of residence, hypertension, diabetes mellitus, and dyslipidemia were stratified in a conditional logistic regression model. ‡ Adjusted model was adjusted for ischemic heart disease, cerebral stroke, Meniere's disease, and head trauma.

In the subgroup analysis according to sex, the OR for BPPV was higher in males (adjusted OR = 1.32, 95% CI = 1.09–1.61, $p = 0.005$, Table 2). There was no increase in the OR for BPPV in female dementia patients.

According to income and region of residence, the subgroups of low income and rural residence showed high OR for BPPV in dementia patients (each of $p < 0.05$). According to the medical histories, the subgroups with histories of hypertension, diabetes, or dyslipidemia, and no histories of ischemic heart disease, stroke, Meniere's disease, or head trauma demonstrated increase in the OR for BPPV in dementia patients (each of $p < 0.05$, Table 3).

Table 3. Subgroup analysis of crude and adjusted odds ratios (95% confidence interval) of BPPV for dementia according to hypertension, diabetes mellitus, dyslipidemia, ischemic heart disease, cerebral stroke, Meniere's disease, and head trauma.

Characteristics	No. of BPPV/ No. of Dementia (%)	No. of BPPV/ No. of Control (%)	Crude †	p-Value	Adjusted †,‡	p-Value	p for Interaction
Non-hypertension (n = 15,590)							
BPPV	112/3118 (3.6)	346/12,472 (2.8)	1.31 (1.05–1.63)	0.016	1.12 (0.89–1.41)	0.327	0.978
Hypertension (n = 41,570)							
BPPV	497/8314 (6.0)	1568/33,256 (4.7)	1.29 (1.16–1.43)	<0.001 *	1.14 (1.03–1.27)	0.016 *	
Non-diabetes mellitus (n = 36,860)							
BPPV	343/7372 (4.7)	1142/29,488 (3.9)	1.21 (1.07–1.37)	0.002 *	1.07 (0.94–1.22)	0.288	0.099
Diabetes mellitus (n = 20,300)							
BPPV	266/4060 (6.6)	772/16,240 (4.8)	1.41 (1.22–1.63)	<0.001 *	1.24 (1.07–1.44)	0.005 *	

Table 3. Cont.

Characteristics	No. of BPPV/ No. of Dementia (%)	No. of BPPV/ No. of Control (%)	ORs for Dementia				p for Interaction
			Crude †	p-Value	Adjusted †,‡	p-Value	
Non-dyslipidemia (n = 39,370)							
BPPV	323/7874 (4.1)	1051/31,496 (3.3)	1.24 (1.09–1.41)	0.001 *	1.11 (0.97–1.27)	0.125	0.500
Dyslipidemia (n = 17,790)							
BPPV	286/3558 (8.0)	863/14,232 (6.1)	1.36 (1.18–1.56)	<0.001 *	1.17 (1.02–1.36)	0.031 *	
Non-ischemic heart disease (n = 49,465)							
BPPV	500/9729 (5.1)	1546/39,736 (3.9)	1.34 (1.21–1.48)	<0.001 *	1.18 (1.06–1.31)	0.003 *	0.107
Ischemic heart disease (n = 7695)							
BPPV	109/1703 (6.4)	368/5992 (6.1)	1.05 (0.84–1.30)	0.693	0.97 (0.77–1.22)	0.781	
Non-cerebral stroke (n = 40,161)							
BPPV	287/5908 (4.9)	1156/34,253 (3.4)	1.46 (1.28–1.67)	<0.001 *	1.46 (1.27–1.67)	<0.001 *	<0.001*
Cerebral stroke (n = 16,999)							
BPPV	322/5524 (5.8)	758/11,475 (6.6)	0.88 (0.77–1.00)	0.052	0.90 (0.79–1.04)	0.146	
Non-Meniere's disease (n = 54,190)							
BPPV	496/10,781 (4.6)	1564/43,409 (3.6)	1.29 (1.16–1.43)	<0.001 *	1.14 (1.02–1.26)	0.020 *	0.934
Meniere's disease (n = 2970)							
BPPV	113/651 (17.4)	350/2319 (15.1)	1.18 (0.94–1.49)	0.160	1.13 (0.89–1.43)	0.318	
Non-head trauma (n = 54,387)							
BPPV	560/10,546 (5.3)	1804/43,841 (4.1)	1.31 (1.19–1.44)	<0.001 *	1.16 (1.05–1.28)	0.005 *	0.163
Head trauma (n = 2773)							
BPPV	49/886 (5.5)	110/1887 (5.8)	0.95 (0.67–1.34)	0.754	0.90 (0.63–1.29)	0.571	

* Odds ratios from a conditional logistic regression model in subgroups according to hypertension, diabetes mellitus, and dyslipidemia, and odds ratios from a unconditional logistic regression model in subgroups according to ischemic heart disease, cerebral stroke, Meniere's disease, and head trauma. Significance at $p < 0.05$, † Age, sex, income, region of residence, hypertension, diabetes mellitus, and dyslipidemia were stratified in a conditional logistic regression model ‡ Adjusted model was adjusted for ischemic heart disease, cerebral stroke, Meniere's disease, and head trauma in a conditional logistic regression model, and age, sex, income, region of residence, hypertension, diabetes mellitus, dyslipidemia, ischemic heart disease, cerebral stroke, Meniere's disease, and head trauma in an unconditional logistic regression model.

4. Discussion

After adjustment for age, sex, income, region of residence, and medical history, the risk of dementia was higher in the BPPV than in the matched control group. Among patients with BPPV, male sex, high income, rural residence, a history of hypertension, diabetes, or dyslipidemia, as well as absence of a history of ischemic heart disease, stroke, Meniere's disease, and head trauma were associated with a high risk of dementia. These findings extend those of previous studies to a larger population with a matched control group.

A previous population cohort study also reported an increased risk of dementia in patients with BPPV (a 1.24-fold higher hazard ratio of dementia in patients with BPPV, 95% confidence interval 1.09–1.40, $p < 0.001$) [11]. However, the control group in the study was matched only for age and sex. Although we adjusted for possible confounders, the effects of unmatched comorbidities on the association between independent and dependent variables cannot be completely excluded [23]. Furthermore, the study included individuals aged ≥20 years, whereas our study included only those aged ≥60 years because dementia is rare in young individuals and usually shows a specific etiology.

BPPV may represent an initial manifestation of degenerative nervous system changes. Vestibular and macular degeneration may lead to otoconial detachment; studies have reported neuronal degenerative changes of the saccular macula in patients with BPPV [24,25]. Degenerative changes in the utricular macula have also been observed in patients with BPPV, who underwent surgery for posterior semicircular canal occlusion [26]. A loss of ganglion cells in the superior or inferior vestibular nerve and saccular ganglion cells, involving approximately 50% and 30%, respectively, of the temporal bone, have been reported in patients with BPPV [27]. Neuronal degeneration is known to affect the phylogenetically older neurons in patients with dementia [28]. The vestibular system is the phylogenetically oldest sensory system [29]; therefore, its degeneration may represent an early or prodromal stage of dementia. Moreover, symptoms of spinning-type vertigo are more prominent than those associated with cognitive impairment; therefore, BPPV tends to be diagnosed earlier than full-blown dementia.

Complications of BPPV, including falls, inactivity, and reduced social activity may contribute to the risk of dementia in patients with BPPV. BPPV is an important contributor to falls in the elderly population [30]. In a retrospective study of elderly patients with BPPV, canalith repositioning therapy was shown to reduce the number of falls [13]. Falls are associated with dementia and serve as an initial presentation in approximately 30% of patients with dementia [31]. Falls may result in traumatic brain injuries, which are shown to be associated with dementia. However, in our subgroup analysis, patients with a history of head trauma did not show an association between BPPV and dementia. Therefore, additional contributors may mediate the association between BPPV and dementia. Comorbidities such as inactivity, anxiety, and depression tend to increase the risk of dementia [32]. Additionally, medications, such as benzodiazepines administered to reduce vertigo or anxiety in patients with BPPV may affect the development of dementia [33]. However, the effects of anxiolytics on subsequent dementia remain controversial [34]. A case–control study reported no definite association between benzodiazepine administration and subsequent dementia [34]. Further studies are warranted to investigate the effects of anxiolytics on dementia.

Shared pathophysiological mechanisms between BPPV and dementia may affect the risks associated with both conditions. A recent study observed that vestibular-system ischemia increased the risk of BPPV [15] and that patients with BPPV showed a high risk of cerebrovascular diseases, including stroke and migraine [15,35]. The association between BPPV and cardiovascular disorders was attributed to ischemia of the feeding arteries of the vestibular system [36]. Vascular compromise in hypertension and heart disease is shown to increase the risk of dementia [37]. In our subgroup analyses based on a history of comorbidities, we observed a definite association between BPPV and an increased risk of dementia in patients with hypertension, diabetes, and dyslipidemia. The high predisposition to both BPPV and dementia may contribute to the higher association between BPPV and dementia. Although we matched and adjusted for confounders, we cannot completely exclude the potential effects of these comorbidities on the association between BPPV and dementia.

Our study also highlighted the higher risk of dementia in men with BPPV. A previous study reported that education level, social activities, and alcohol consumption interact with sex to affect cognitive function [38] and may also play a role in the sex-based differences in the risk of dementia in patients with BPPV. Furthermore, in this study, high income and rural residence affected the association between BPPV and the increased risk of dementia. Access to healthcare is invariably affected by income levels. This study was based on health-claims data; therefore, it is reasonable to conclude that clinical visits for evaluation of BPPV may be higher in patients with a high income.

The present study was based on nationwide representative data, the validity of which was verified by a previous study [21]. The National Health Interview Survey data include all Korean citizens, without exception; therefore, there were no missing participants. The control group was randomly selected and matched for age, sex, income, region of residence, and a medical history of hypertension, diabetes, and dyslipidemia. We included income and region of residence because these factors tend to determine the availability of healthcare.

Following are the limitations of our study. BPPV was diagnosed by a physician in patients who were treated at least twice for the condition. However, BPPV was not categorized based on severity and subtypes. Various pathophysiological conditions, including cupulolithiasis, canal switch, and re-entry phenomenon are associated with BPPV [39]. The diagnosis of BPPV could be inaccurate, particularly in elderly patients owing to the vague history and difficulty in physical examination in this population [40]. Positional nystagmus of central origin may also manifest as BPPV [41]. Reportedly, approximately 97.5% of central positional nystagmus manifests as an atypical direction of nystagmus observed during the Dix–Hallpike maneuver; however, central positional nystagmus secondary to cerebellar or brainstem involvement may mimic and be misdiagnosed as BPPV [41]. The diagnosis of BPPV may be missed by general physicians; BPPV is more accurately diagnosed by otoneurologists than by general practitioners. Compared with healthy controls, patients with comorbidities are more likely to be diagnosed with BPPV owing to frequent clinical visits. Although we adjusted for several potential confounders, we did not consider a few others, including body mass index, smoking status, alcohol consumption, physical inactivity, social isolation, education level, and hearing loss. The dementia group in this study was selected based on the International Classification of Diseases, Tenth Revision, Clinical Modification codes and a history of treatment with more than one therapeutic intervention for the condition. The prevalence of dementia assumed in this study was comparable with that reported by the Central Dementia Center of Korea. However, data from the Health Insurance Review and Assessment Service National Patient Sample do not include details regarding the severity of dementia; additionally, we could not determine semicircular-canal involvement and eventual recovery from BPPV.

5. Conclusions

BPPV was related with an increased risk of dementia in patients ≥ 60 years of age. This association of BPPV with dementia was valid in patients with male sex, low income, rural residence, and medical histories of hypertension, diabetes, and dyslipidemia. The possible links of BPPV with dementia need to be considered when managing patients with BPPV.

Author Contributions: H.G.C. designed the study; D.M.Y., C.M. and H.G.C. analyzed the data; S.Y.K. and H.G.C. drafted and revised the paper; and H.G.C. drew the figures. All authors have read and agreed to the published version of the manuscript.

Funding: This work was supported in part by research grants (NRF-2018-R1D1A1A02085328, 2020R1A2C4002594 and 2021-R1C1C100498611) from the National Research Foundation (NRF) of Korea. The APC was funded by NRF-2021-R1C1C100498611.

Institutional Review Board Statement: The Ethics Committee of Hallym University (2014-I148) approved the use of the data. The need for written informed consent was waived by the Institutional Review Board.

Informed Consent Statement: Written informed consent was waived by the Institutional Review Board.

Data Availability Statement: Releasing of the data by the researcher is not legally permitted. All data are available from the database of the Korea Center for Disease Control and Prevention. The Korea Center for Disease Control and Prevention allows data access, at a particular cost, for any researcher who promises to follow the research ethics. The data of this article can be downloaded from the website after agreeing to follow the research ethics.

Conflicts of Interest: The authors declare no conflict of interest.

References

1. Harun, A.; Oh, E.S.; Bigelow, R.T.; Studenski, S.; Agrawal, Y. Vestibular Impairment in Dementia. *Otol. Neurotol.* **2016**, *37*, 1137–1142. [CrossRef]
2. Lee, H.-W.; Lim, Y.-H.; Kim, S.-H. Dizziness in patients with cognitive impairment. *J. Vestib. Res.* **2020**, *30*, 17–23. [CrossRef]
3. Smith, P.F. Why dizziness is likely to increase the risk of cognitive dysfunction and dementia in elderly adults. *N. Z. Med. J.* **2020**, *133*, 112–127.
4. Liu, P.; Zheng, Y.; King, J.; Darlington, C.; Smith, P. Long-term changes in hippocampal n-methyl-d-aspartate receptor subunits following unilateral vestibular damage in rat. *Neuroscience* **2003**, *117*, 965–970. [CrossRef]

5. Brandt, T.; Schautzer, F.; Hamilton, D.A.; Brüning, R.; Markowitsch, H.J.; Kalla, R.; Darlington, C.; Smith, P.; Strupp, M. Vestibular loss causes hippocampal atrophy and impaired spatial memory in humans. *Brain* 2005, *128*, 2732–2741. [CrossRef]
6. Batuecas-Caletrío, Á.; Trinidad-Ruiz, G.; Zschaeck, C.; del Pozo de Dios, J.C.; Gil, L.D.T.; Martín-Sánchez, V.; Martin-Sanz, E. Benign Paroxysmal Positional Vertigo in the Elderly. *Gerontology* 2013, *59*, 408–412. [CrossRef]
7. Cho, E.I.; White, J.A. Positional Vertigo: As Occurs Across All Age Groups. *Otolaryngol. Clin. North Am.* 2011, *44*, 347–360. [CrossRef]
8. Shim, D.B. Treatment of Benign Paroxysmal Positional Vertigo: An Approach Considering Patients' Convenience. *Clin. Exp. Otorhinolaryngol.* 2020, *13*, 320–321. [CrossRef]
9. Ribeiro, K.F.; Oliveira, B.S.; Freitas, R.V.; Ferreira, L.M.; Deshpande, N.; Guerra, R. Effectiveness of Otolith Repositioning Maneuvers and Vestibular Rehabilitation exercises in elderly people with Benign Paroxysmal Positional Vertigo: A systematic review. *Braz. J. Otorhinolaryngol.* 2018, *84*, 109–118. [CrossRef]
10. Lee, H.J.; Jeon, E.-J.; Lee, D.-H.; Seo, J.-H. Therapeutic Efficacy of the Modified Epley Maneuver with a Pillow Under the Shoulders. *Clin. Exp. Otorhinolaryngol.* 2020, *13*, 376–380. [CrossRef]
11. Lo, M.-H.; Lin, C.-L.; Chuang, E.; Chuang, T.-Y.; Kao, C.-H. Association of dementia in patients with benign paroxysmal positional vertigo. *Acta Neurol. Scand.* 2017, *135*, 197–203. [CrossRef]
12. Montero-Odasso, M.; Speechley, M. Falls in Cognitively Impaired Older Adults: Implications for Risk Assessment and Prevention. *J. Am. Geriatr. Soc.* 2018, *66*, 367–375. [CrossRef]
13. Ganança, F.F.; Gazzola, J.M.; Ganança, C.F.; Caovilla, H.H.; Ganança, M.M.; Cruz, O.L.M. Elderly falls associated with benign paroxysmal positional vertigo. *Braz. J. Otorhinolaryngol.* 2010, *76*, 113–120. [CrossRef]
14. Von Brevern, M.; Radtke, A.; Lezius, F.; Feldmann, M.; Ziese, T.; Lempert, T.; Neuhauser, H. Epidemiology of benign paroxysmal positional vertigo: A population based study. *J. Neurol. Neurosurg. Psychiatry* 2006, *78*, 710–715. [CrossRef]
15. Ekao, C.-L.; Cheng, Y.-Y.; Eleu, H.-B.; Echen, T.-J.; Ema, H.-I.; Echen, J.-W.; Elin, S.-J.; Echan, R.-C. Increased Risk of Ischemic Stroke in Patients with Benign Paroxysmal Positional Vertigo: A 9-Year Follow-Up Nationwide Population Study in Taiwan. *Front. Aging Neurosci.* 2014, *6*, 108. [CrossRef]
16. Wolters, F.J.; Segufa, R.A.; Darweesh, S.K.; Bos, D.; Ikram, M.A.; Sabayan, B.; Hofman, A.; Sedaghat, S. Coronary heart disease, heart failure, and the risk of dementia: A systematic review and meta-analysis. *Alzheimer's Dement.* 2018, *14*, 1493–1504. [CrossRef] [PubMed]
17. Kim, H.M.; Lee, Y.-H.; Han, K.; Lee, B.-W.; Kang, E.S.; Kim, J.; Cha, B.-S. Impact of diabetes mellitus and chronic liver disease on the incidence of dementia and all-cause mortality among patients with dementia. *Medicine* 2017, *96*, e8753. [CrossRef] [PubMed]
18. Lourenco, J.; Serrano, A.; Santos-Silva, A.; Gomes, M.; Afonso, C.; Freitas, P.; Paul, C.; Costa, E. Cardiovascular Risk Factors Are Correlated with Low Cognitive Function among Older Adults Across Europe Based on The SHARE Database. *Aging Dis.* 2018, *9*, 90–101. [CrossRef]
19. Mendez, M.F. Early-Onset Alzheimer Disease. *Neurol. Clin.* 2017, *35*, 263–281. [CrossRef]
20. Kim, S.Y.; Min, C.; Yoo, D.M.; Chang, J.; Lee, H.-J.; Park, B.; Choi, H.G. Hearing Impairment Increases Economic Inequality. *Clin. Exp. Otorhinolaryngol.* 2021, *14*, 278–286. [CrossRef]
21. Lee, J.; Lee, J.S.; Park, S.-H.; Shin, S.A.; Kim, K. Cohort Profile: The National Health Insurance Service–National Sample Cohort (NHIS-NSC), South Korea. *Int. J. Epidemiol.* 2016, *46*, 319. [CrossRef]
22. National Health Insurance Sharing Service. Available online: http://nhiss.nhis.or.kr/ (accessed on 1 January 2016).
23. Kim, S.Y.; Sim, S.; Kim, H.-J.; Choi, H.G. Sudden sensory neural hearing loss is not predictive of myocardial infarction: A longitudinal follow-up study using a national sample cohort. *Sci. Rep.* 2018, *8*, 1–7. [CrossRef] [PubMed]
24. Eryaman, E.; Oz, I.D.; Ozker, B.Y.; Erbek, S.S. Evaluation of vestibular evoked myogenic potentials during benign paroxysmal positional vertigo attacks; neuroepithelial degeneration? *B-ENT* 2012, *8*, 247–250.
25. Yang, W.S.; Kim, S.H.; Lee, J.D.; Lee, W.-S. Clinical Significance of Vestibular Evoked Myogenic Potentials in Benign Paroxysmal Positional Vertigo. *Otol. Neurotol.* 2008, *29*, 1162–1166. [CrossRef] [PubMed]
26. Parnes, L.S.; McClure, J.A. Free-Floating Endolymph Particles: A new operative finding during posterior semicircular canal occlusion. *Laryngoscope* 1992, *102*, 988–992. [CrossRef]
27. Gacek, R.R. Pathology of Benign Paroxysmal Positional Vertigo Revisited. *Ann. Otol. Rhinol. Laryngol.* 2003, *112*, 574–582. [CrossRef]
28. Lyness, S.; Zarow, C.; Chui, H.C. Neuron loss in key cholinergic and aminergic nuclei in Alzheimer disease: A meta-analysis. *Neurobiol. Aging* 2002, *24*, 1–23. [CrossRef]
29. Nandi, R.; Luxon, L.M. Development and assessment of the vestibular system. *Int. J. Audiol.* 2008, *47*, 566–577. [CrossRef] [PubMed]
30. Abbott, J.; Tomassen, S.; Lane, L.; Bishop, K.; Thomas, N. Assessment for benign paroxysmal positional vertigo in medical patients admitted with falls in a district general hospital. *Clin. Med.* 2016, *16*, 335–338. [CrossRef]
31. Buchner, D.M.; Larson, E.B. Falls and fractures in patients with Alzheimer-type dementia. *JAMA* 1987, *257*, 1492–1495. [CrossRef]
32. Peluso, É.T.P.; Quintana, M.I.; Ganança, F.F. Anxiety and depressive disorders in elderly with chronic dizziness of vestibular origin. *Braz. J. Otorhinolaryngol.* 2016, *82*, 209–214. [CrossRef] [PubMed]
33. Jacqmin-Gadda, H.; Guillet, F.; Mathieu, C.; Helmer, C.; Pariente, A.; Joly, P. Impact of benzodiazepine consumption reduction on future burden of dementia. *Sci. Rep.* 2020, *10*, 1–9. [CrossRef] [PubMed]

34. Osler, M.; Jørgensen, M.B. Associations of Benzodiazepines, Z-Drugs, and Other Anxiolytics with Subsequent Dementia in Patients With Affective Disorders: A Nationwide Cohort and Nested Case-Control Study. *Am. J. Psychiatry* **2020**, *177*, 497–505. [CrossRef] [PubMed]
35. Chu, C.-H.; Liu, C.-J.; Lin, L.-Y.; Chen, T.-J.; Wang, S.-J. Migraine is associated with an increased risk for benign paroxysmal positional vertigo: A nationwide population-based study. *J. Headache Pain* **2015**, *16*, 1–7. [CrossRef]
36. Zhang, D.; Zhang, S.; Zhang, H.; Xu, Y.; Fu, S.; Yu, M.; Ji, P. Evaluation of vertebrobasilar artery changes in patients with benign paroxysmal positional vertigo. *NeuroReport* **2013**, *24*, 741–745. [CrossRef]
37. Luchsinger, J.A.; Reitz, C.; Honig, L.S.; Tang, M.X.; Shea, S.; Mayeux, R. Aggregation of vascular risk factors and risk of incident Alzheimer disease. *Neurology* **2005**, *65*, 545–551. [CrossRef] [PubMed]
38. Kim, M.; Park, J.-M. Factors affecting cognitive function according to gender in community-dwelling elderly individuals. *Epidemiol. Health* **2017**, *39*, e2017054. [CrossRef]
39. Priola, R.S.F.; Lorusso, F.; Immordino, A.; Dispenza, F. Complex forms of benign paroxysmal positional vertigo. In *Dizziness: Prevalence, Risk Factors and Management*; Nova Publisher: Hauppauge, NY, USA, 2021; pp. 117–149.
40. Balatsouras, D.G.; Fassolis, G.K.; Moukos, A.; Apris, A. Benign paroxysmal positional vertigo in the elderly: Current insights. *Clin. Interv. Aging* **2018**, *13*, 2251–2266. [CrossRef]
41. Macdonald, N.K.; Kaski, D.; Saman, Y.; Sulaiman, A.A.-S.; Anwer, A.; Bamiou, D.-E. Central Positional Nystagmus: A Systematic Literature Review. *Front. Neurol.* **2017**, *8*. [CrossRef]

MDPI
St. Alban-Anlage 66
4052 Basel
Switzerland
www.mdpi.com

International Journal of Environmental Research and Public Health Editorial Office
E-mail: ijerph@mdpi.com
www.mdpi.com/journal/ijerph

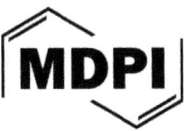

Disclaimer/Publisher's Note: The statements, opinions and data contained in all publications are solely those of the individual author(s) and contributor(s) and not of MDPI and/or the editor(s). MDPI and/or the editor(s) disclaim responsibility for any injury to people or property resulting from any ideas, methods, instructions or products referred to in the content.

www.ingramcontent.com/pod-product-compliance
Lightning Source LLC
LaVergne TN
LVHW070551100526
838202LV00012B/440